Evaluating Improvement and Implementation for Health

Evaluating Improvement and Implementation for Health

John Øvretveit

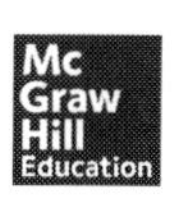

Open University Press

Open University Press
McGraw-Hill Education
McGraw-Hill House
Shoppenhangers Road
Maidenhead
Berkshire
England
SL6 2QL

email: enquiries@openup.co.uk
world wide web: www.openup.co.uk

and Two Penn Plaza, New York, NY 10121-2289, USA

First published 2014

A catalogue record of this book is available from the British Library

ISBN-13: 978-0-33-524277-1 (pb)
ISBN-10: 0-33-524277-4 (pb)
eISBN: 978-0-33-524278-8

Library of Congress Cataloging-in-Publication Data
CIP data applied for

Typesetting and e-book compilations by
RefineCatch Limited, Bungay, Suffolk

Praise for this book

"For anyone looking for a readable and complete introduction to evaluation, the search ends at* Evaluating Improvement and Implementation for Health *by John Øvretveit. It provides an overview of evaluation in action for making better decisions about how to improve health outcomes for individuals, communities, and nations. The emphasis on including assessments of implementation as a necessary part of any evaluation is refreshing and the examples throughout the book illuminate the concepts and pique the reader's curiosity right to the end. Reading this book is time well spent."

Dean L. Fixsen, Ph.D., University of North Carolina at Chapel Hill, Senior Scientist, FPG Child Development Institute, Co-Director, National Implementation Research Network, USA

Contents

Foreword

As the author notes by quoting a famous evaluator, one important issue is not whether we evaluate, but how well we do it. As health care systems around the world struggle with the common challenges of aging populations, rapidly rising expenditures and the growing prevalence of chronic illnesses, there is enormous enthusiasm and a growing marketplace for innovations that promise to address our current dilemmas – preferably painlessly. However, too many interventions are taken up without proper testing, and only later do leaders, clinicians and the public learn that the gap between ideas and effective implementation can be a chasm, e.g., the 'new new thing' is less effective than the enthusiasts suggested, there are safety or cost issues or we haven't thought through a number of issues such as capacity to customize for a particular set of circumstances or the time frame for achieving success. Rodgers famously observed in his classic book, *Diffusion of Innovation*, that the loss in effectiveness that occurs when interventions are applied to new settings has received far too little scrutiny. With the rapid growth in innovations and market opportunities, we desperately need independent evaluation to guide our decisions about which to adopt, how quickly and when.

This is important for those allocating financial resources through insurance to pay for some interventions and services which may be taking resources from other more effective ones, as well as those leading large health care systems struggling with 'make or buy' issues. It is also important, as this book observes, to evaluate how we implement already-evaluated improvements in different settings and contexts. When evaluation shows what may be effective, we may lose lives or large amounts of resources because take-up is slow and variable, even when people agree about what is a better way. 'Implementation' suggests a straightforward translation from evaluation research to practice, but it is rarely as simple as that. We need to use evaluation also to learn which of the different implementation methods and infrastructures are effective for enabling take-up of proven improvements, and how to customize the applications without losing fidelity to the goals of intervention.

One reason many interventions and changes are not evaluated is because they may not be amenable to evaluation through experimental methods. This does not mean that they cannot be evaluated. There are a range of designs, which, if properly chosen and applied, can provide actionable knowledge. The perfect can be the enemy of the good, so long as the good comes with a clear statement of the limitations of the findings. The ethics of evaluation include evaluators spelling out these limitations, as they often know best the strengths and weaknesses of their findings, as well as taking a properly skeptical and neutral attitude to the intervention. Moreover, far too many examples of dramatic improvements in care delivery led by charismatic leaders in one setting that failed to succeed in others underscore the value of a skeptical belief system.

Another reason why innovations are not evaluated is that there are so many treatments, service models and policies under development or use. Deciding which to evaluate is not an issue the book addresses, but one which I faced daily in my work as Director of AHRQ. An especially challenging issue for evaluators and improvement research sponsors concerns the timing of when to evaluate and how to assess the specific context in which the intervention is being tested. Should all improvement efforts be tested first for efficacy, or can development and implementation proceed concurrently? By showing the range of methods and interventions which can be evaluated, and the valuable actionable information which evaluation can provide, this book might be viewed as a 'marketing pitch' for evaluation. It is not, however, a prescriptive set of rules that makes decisions foolproof. Rather, it makes the decisions of those funding evaluations more difficult as we cannot quickly eliminate evaluation proposals because they do not use experimental methods. We and our proposal reviewers need to know more about what different evaluation methods can and cannot deliver, and why. We also need to consider whether more resources should be given to evaluations of non-medical interventions when less rigorous but more relevant evaluation methods can provide useful information to decision-makers and implementers. As the funding environment for care delivery becomes more constrained, public and private sector decision-makers will increasingly confront questions such as what percentage of a pharmaceutical budget is worth investing in evaluating interventions to enhance precise identification of those most likely to benefit from new treatments and to help those individuals adhere to the treatment at hand. Or how would reductions in cost sharing impact individuals' ability to obtain and use needed services?

There are initiatives in the USA and elsewhere which are leading to more relevant, responsive and rigorous evaluations. At the same time there are ongoing debates regarding the best way to approach the question 'how do we know?', most notably in relation to assessing the impact of expanding access to health care, but also with respect to understanding which innovations in finance and delivery have the potential to be adopted as future policy for all. This book is to be welcomed for its wide-ranging overview and introduction to the many approaches to evaluation. It can be used by non-researchers to learn about different evaluation methods, some of which may be more suitable to their questions than other methods.

Carolyn M. Clancy, MD
Former Director,
Agency for Healthcare Research and Quality (AHRQ) (2003 – 2013)

Acknowledgements

I would like to acknowledge the assistance of four people who have been important to me and have enabled me to write this book: Mats Brommels, Director of LIME at the Karolinska Institute, who not only granted me the time to devote to this book, but who also has greatly influenced me by his practical and thoughtful approaches to ways to make a difference for patients. Second, Dr Brian Mittman, a leader in implementation research and one of the founders of the journal, *Implementation Science*, and from whom I have learned so much over the years about this new and growing multidiscipline. And, finally, two of the founders of improvement science, but also two people, who, by their humanity and integrity, have had a great influence on me when the going got hard and I wondered if it was worth it: Don Berwick and Brent James.

Part I Introduction: Concepts

The basic ideas

Many people providing services and making policy have to make decisions – that's what they are paid for. Their decisions can be informed by evaluation if the evaluation is designed and carried out in the right way: by matching the users' question to the design and working with them on the evaluation. This is the theme of the book and, in my view, the future for relevant but also rigorous evaluation. Being relevant does not mean an evaluation cannot be scientific and published: indeed, it is not relevant if it does not use systematic and objective methods. The perfect can be the enemy of the good and better some knowledge than none, as long as the evaluator makes clear the limitations.

Part I introduces 'user-centred evaluation' and the 'matching' theme. We begin Chapter 1 by asking 'Would prescribing pets be cost-effective?' In my view, paying for an 'animal companion', as they say in the USA, for single older people who might consider such an idea, would improve health and reduce the costs of healthcare. But that's only my view. What is the evidence? How would we find out? We introduce the idea that some evaluations give more certainty than others, and that you often get what you pay for. If you are prepared to wait some time and pay evaluators a large sum of money, then you can increase the certainty of the evaluation. But are there less expensive and quicker evaluations which give 'good enough' knowledge to inform action? Chapters 1 and 2 introduce the distinction between an intervention and what is done to implement it, and how we can evaluate implementation approaches.

Chapter 3 gives a 'quick start' guide to the eight steps for carrying out an evaluation. If you understand this, then you might not need to read Chapter 2. This explains evaluation concepts and is a bit boring because it has to be fairly abstract. But the chapter does use an example to illustrate the ideas: an evaluation to find out if 'active multidisciplinary rehabilitation' is more effective than 'traditional primary care rehabilitation'.

Chapter 4 is about pictures. If you cannot draw it, you do not understand the design. The chapter shows how pictures with a timeline help to think through the most important parts of the evaluation and communicate this to others. It describes three types of design: (1) experimental and quasi-experimental; (2) observational; and (3) action approaches to evaluation.

Part II is all about real evaluations in these three categories of experimental, observational and action evaluations. Each chapter in this Part takes three examples and discusses their strengths and weaknesses and asks: 'Is this the best match between the users' question and the design, given the constraints of the evaluation?'

1 Evaluating health interventions, improvements and their implementation

Introduction

Pets for older people are said to improve health and might reduce their use of healthcare. Do they? Would prescribing pets be cost-effective? What about prescribing a 'Fitbit' – a coin-sized device you put in your pocket which tells you how many steps you took today? Evaluations answer these questions, but some designs answer them better than others. The aim of this book is to give those new to evaluation an overview of when to carry out or buy an evaluation, as well to give researchers a guide to different evaluation approaches.

Chapter 5, which opens Part II of the book, does not show how to evaluate whether prescribing pets is cost-effective. But it does show an example evaluation of prescribing exercise. In so doing, it demonstrates evaluation principles and methods, which is how this book aims to help you better to understand evaluation and to excite you with the possibilities – through examples. Those running courses on evaluation can use these examples and the questions as case studies for groups. Chapter 11 shows how to evaluate the return on investment of pet-prescribing and how to assess if there is a business case for this intervention. The Fitbit is one of the digital applications which are revolutionizing healthcare, most have not been evaluated – the subject of Chapter 12.

But if it works, what is the best way to implement it? What is the best way to enable doctors to prescribe pets or Fitbits, or to enable patients to get one and live with one? Implementing a treatment, a change, or a policy can be challenging, even if it is a proven improvement elsewhere. There are methods and strategies which are more or less effective in enabling patients or providers and others to take up, adopt and adapt an intervention. The rapidly growing science of implementation gives us methods for evaluating these strategies and for assessing which ones are best for which interventions in which situations – the subject of Chapter 10, which opens Part III on special topics.

Improvements in health, and sometimes lower costs, come from better treatments and from better healthcare. The other chapters in Part II demonstrate how to evaluate treatment interventions as well as interventions to providers, for example, to help them use treatments appropriately or to help them redesign their clinic. The chapters in Part II are grouped into types of intervention. That is because the book aims to be user-focused. Readers may want to see quickly how to evaluate a particular type of intervention or service. The examples in Part II show the reader how to do this, but not only for interventions to patients or to providers. Evaluations are also needed of larger-scale changes to health systems and to communities. Health improvements come from population health interventions, such as health education, health promotion and public health services which are not healthcare services. They are often more difficult to evaluate and need modifications to the traditional evaluation methods as well as new methods. This is why a separate chapter, Chapter 9, is given over to showing how these can be evaluated.

Do I need to read Part I?

Do you expect an author to agree you do not read one-third of their book? Try any chapter in Parts II and III and see how you go: most of these chapters draw on the Part I chapters. You may know enough already not to need the details of design, the evaluation concepts and the steps for carrying out an evaluation described in Part I.

Chapter 1 also considers how evaluation is breaking down the separation between research and practice through the idea of the learning health system (Etheredge 2007; IOM 2007; Academy Health 2012) and real-time research. How many of my patients are using treatment Y and what are their outcomes, compared to those using treatment X? The digital revolution is making it possible for practitioners to do real-time evaluations and answer these questions with the patient in the room. Data from the patient's electronic medical records and other databases can quickly be searched and analysed using modern software to show in seconds the answers to what were traditionally two- or three-year research evaluations. When the results are presented to providers and patients together, as one Swedish system does, we also enable self-care (Øvretveit et al. 2013).

Common questions answered by evaluations

- Does it work? (Better than what?, In what respect?, Are there risks?, How certain are we of the risks?)
- Who does it work best for? (Generalizability?)
- What was the experience like for patients?
- How much does it cost? (Does the money come from my budget, and who gets the savings?)
- Are the methods they used to enable uptake (or implement) the intervention effective?
- Did this change give what the politician or manager said it would?

Improvement and implementation

Is it really an improvement?

'Improvement' suggests that the intervention has already been found to improve health or healthcare in some way. But to call something an improvement before it has been evaluated is not strictly correct – it is a *potential* improvement. One of the aims of evaluation is to find out if an intervention or change really is an improvement, in one or more respects. And immediately we are plunged into controversy, which is inherent to evaluation: it might improve patient satisfaction but it costs more. Some will not see this as an improvement, or one worth the costs. The point being that evaluations are limited, there are conflicting perspectives and needs, and not all of these needs can be met by one evaluation. Evaluations are only able to assess a few results of an intervention. There will be other results which are unknown but which actually may be significant (e.g. do the long-term effects of the medication increase the risk of cancer?). There will also be many people whose questions are not answered by an evaluation (e.g. is it worth the cost?).

What are 'health improvements'?

- Some health interventions are to communities.
- Some healthcare interventions are to individual providers or healthcare service organizations. (These are intended to improve the provider practice or organization in some way, one improvement being to enable them to provide better health services to patients or communities.)
- Some health treatments and services are to patients.

Do improvements need to be implemented?

It is also about how to evaluate how interventions are implemented: how they are 'taken up' by patients, providers, organizations or communities. Many evaluations are done in one place and with one patient group, and time and effort are put into properly implementing the intervention so that it then can be evaluated. If it works, and others want to implement it, they want to know what was done to implement it and if it would work for their patients or communities, where the circumstances are different. Evaluations need to describe and consider how they enabled the uptake of the intervention, not just if it worked.

We are generally cautious about changing what we do. We need to be convinced and motivated that the treatment or new way is much better, if we are to expend the time and energy to change habits and ways of working. Even if a treatment or change has been proved to be effective, it will need special action and effort for it to be taken up by a patient, provider, organization or community. Usually a strategy, structure and support are needed, unless it is one of those rare interventions which are taken up without assistance.

The point is that evaluations are also needed regarding how treatments or changes are implemented. Implementation evaluation is a new subject in healthcare, in part because traditional medical evaluation research focused on whether an intervention worked. A traditional controlled trial evaluation expends considerable time and effort to ensure the intervention is fully applied (e.g. the patients take the drug, or the providers undergo the training) and focuses on whether it then makes a difference. The implementation is a tedious step to overcome so as to allow the real evaluation to take place.

But supposing the intervention is very effective and others want to adopt it? Do they have the resources used in the controlled trial to implement it? Of interest to others is what the evaluators did to ensure the intervention was fully implemented, and what they would need to do to implement successfully in their own situation. Controlled trial 'outcome' evaluations often give limited information about this. Some have used process evaluations, carried out in parallel to the trial, to discover how an intervention was implemented in different places and on different patients where the trial protocol cannot enforce implementation. More information on this is given in Chapter 10.

Monitoring, measurement and evaluation

To monitor a treatment, a service, a programme or a policy requires the use of different data at different times to check and decide if action is needed. Monitoring may or may not use measurement. Measurement provides data numerically. The numerical data may be given by a device that measures blood pressure. Or a rating scale such as 'Please rate your understanding of the information the nurse provided' on a scale of 0–10, where 0 = could not understand and 10 = very easy to understand. Note that a question which is more 'actionable' for the nurse or manager is one which is more specific and behavioural, e.g. 'Did the nurse give you any information about how to contact her if you needed to?' But providing information which directs to action is another point, and not one we will pursue here.

Is measuring patient understanding using this method of asking them to express their experience by a number really an evaluation? It is true that this is asking patients to judge the value of the service on this dimension. But I would suggest that data from one measure are not a real evaluation, because there is no explicit and systematic comparison. It would need at least two measurement points to be an evaluation of what the nurse did or what a service provided – either now compared to last month, or now compared to what people say about another service at this time.

If there is no comparison, is there is no evaluation?

Humans are creatures who automatically make comparisons. We are wired instinctively to use comparison to make judgements which help us decide on action. It is an evolutionary feature which has helped us to learn and survive as a species this far. Evaluation is making a systematic and objective comparison.

Humans are very quick to make judgements. Honed over thousands of years, the ability quickly to judge if we could eat an animal, or if it would eat us, was imprinted on those who survived. More thoughtful evaluation is more complex and slow to judge. We have to be careful to find the right information and to use it in the right way in order to make our value judgement. We are clearer about what is important to us: our criteria of valuation, and we are using *systematic evaluation*.

We also have to be careful about how we make a link between our value judgement and what action to take. In systematic evaluation the usual approach is to separate the collection of information (the task of the 'evaluator') from judging value and acting (the task of the 'user' of the evaluation). Other differences from everyday evaluation are the evaluator's careful definition of what is to be evaluated, and of the information needed, as well as his or her careful selection and use of methods to collect and analyse the information.

Systematic evaluation is also complex in that the evaluator has to know a range of methods and approaches so as to be able to choose the best method for the purpose of the evaluation. We do not use methods such as participant observation and grounded theory to find information about the cost of home care in comparison to hospital care, but we may use these methods if the aim is to find out how patients and carers judge or make use of these types of care. Ideally, the evaluator has to be able to use a variety of methods, or at least to know which method is best for the purpose of the evaluation. Ideally, those sponsoring and managing an evaluation should be able to make an independent judgement about what can and cannot be expected from a proposed evaluation, and whether other methods would be more cost-effective for what they need.

What is evaluation?

I realized the word 'evaluation' meant different things to different people when my American brother-in-law said we were going to the shop to 'evaluate the TVs'. He had decided to buy a new one and wanted to compare them. There are 142 different definitions of evaluation. I still have not found one better than this:

> Evaluation is making a comparative assessment of the value of something, using systematically collected and analysed data, in order to decide how to act.

A slightly longer definition highlights the important features of evaluation:

> Evaluation is attributing value to something, by gathering reliable and valid information about it in a systematic way, and by making comparisons, for the purposes of making more informed decisions or understanding causal mechanisms and generalizable principles.
>
> (Øvretveit 1998)

Let us unpack this second definition, teasing out the meanings of the separate parts:

> . . . *attributing value to something* . . .

The something is a thing or process, the value of which we are judging. It is often called an intervention or the change that was introduced (as opposed to a change in subjects which may have resulted from the intervention, which is one outcome). The interventions we consider later are health treatments and services for patients. We also consider changes to individual providers (clinicians) such as training, or changes to healthcare organizations such as a new financing method. Later the book looks at intervention changes called policies, and programmes, which intervene with effect on communities or populations.

Is a drug treatment a very different intervention from a 5-year health promotion programme for a population? Are the interventions and changes in each of these categories very different in their nature and complexity? Because of the differences in these interventions, with various subjects of change, in Part II we consider how evaluation designs are modified to evaluate these different types of intervention change, and why some designs cannot be used.

Some interventions and changes are easier to define than others: a standard drug treatment can be specified and does not change, while a healthcare reform or quality improvement intervention is difficult to specify and may change as it is implemented, even if we try to keep it standardized. Defining or specifying what we are evaluating is important because we want to be sure exactly what it is that we are judging the value of. Even treatments can be difficult to define exactly, as we will see when we look at 'alternative' treatments such as aromatherapy and homeopathy.

Giving an exact definition often becomes more difficult as we move from biophysical systems to social systems such as services delivery organizations, and then to 'higher-level' social systems when we look at a health policy such as a ban on smoking which is implemented across health and other sectors. Then there are health reforms, which are truly volatile interventions. We will see that evaluators need to spend some time defining the intervention or change, and that the only purpose of some evaluations is to get a clearer description of an intervention or change.

Note also that the term 'intervention' comes from the Latin words 'inter' and 'venire', which means 'to come between' what otherwise would have happened. Without the drug, the patient's physiology would have followed process X and the patient would have experienced Y. If the drug were an intervention, then it 'came between' these processes.

Strictly speaking, the evaluation is to find out if there was an intervention: did the change alter anything? Similarly, what are referred to as 'outcomes' may not necessarily 'come out' of the intervention: outcome evaluations have to find out how much the intervention and not something else caused what are said to be the outcomes.

If it's all about data collection, how do we judge value?

If we are able to define the intervention or change, how then do we then judge its value, or 'attribute' value to it? The first point is that it is the 'users' of the evaluation who judge the value of the intervention, that is, the patients, the providers, the politicians, the managers, the citizens, and others. Strictly speaking, evaluators do not judge value. They simply collect, analyse and present information. The information that they collect and the way they present it are designed to concentrate on certain things, which some, or all, users think are important for them to be able to judge the value of the intervention.

The definition given above includes 'attributing value' because it aims to encompass the whole process of evaluation and to draw attention to the part that users play in evaluations, rather than keeping this separate. I think that there is something lacking in a definition and understanding of evaluation which does not include valuation. This definition recognizes the process of valuation and this book shows how values enter into most parts of the evaluation process.

... gathering reliable and valid information about it in a systematic way ...

The second part of the definition shows one way in which an evaluation helps users to attribute value: the evaluation presents them with information about the intervention which is reliable and valid and has been gathered by evaluators in a systematic way for the purposes of judging value. This distinguishes evaluation from journalism, where the journalist does not use the same rigorous methods. What, then, is the difference between evaluation and other types of research, which also give valid and reliable information about an intervention?

... by making comparisons ...

Comparison is the main way in which evaluation helps users to attribute value, and, together with valuation, is what distinguishes evaluation from some other types of research. Different types of evaluation carry out different types of comparison:

- they compare the state of one or more people, populations or organizations before an intervention to their state after the intervention;
- they compare the needs of people or populations before an intervention to their needs after an intervention;
- they compare one group of people to another group who undergo a different intervention or none at all, to see if the exposure to the intervention affects the exposed group in some way;
- they compare what is done to a set of standards or guidelines (e.g. perform an audit);
- they compare the objectives of the intervention to the actual achievements.

We can only judge value if we make a comparison. Many evaluations use 'value criteria' to help make the comparison, or only one criterion, such as symptom relief, cost or the number of eligible people using a service. In 'before and after' evaluations, the criterion is the before and after measure. In a two-group evaluation model, the criterion is used to measure the state of the two groups. In the other types above, the criterion is the objectives, standards or guidelines.

Where do value criteria come from?

A value criterion, such as patient experience, shapes one set of data we collect, and gives one of the ways we judge the value of the intervention. Value criteria come from users of the evaluation. Or they are predefined (e.g. established standards which value certain features), and users agree to adopt them to help them judge the value of the intervention or change.

We should recognize, though, that people judge the value of the intervention or change using many criteria. Many judgements are made subconsciously or from half-formed criteria, and are different for different people and interest groups. Evaluators may help people to clarify the criteria of valuation which they want to use. This point – that an evaluation makes a limited comparison using limited criteria – takes us to the next part of the definition:

. . . for the purposes of making more informed decisions . . .

Examples of decisions are, whether or when to use a treatment, how to improve a service, or whether to limit or discontinue it. Others may be about how to set up other similar services or whether to abandon, extend or modify a policy, or how best to implement an already proven intervention.

We need to add the phrase '*than they would otherwise do*' to the phrase '*more informed decisions*'. People do not need an evaluation to judge the value of something and to decide how to act. Very few treatments, services or other interventions have been or ever will be evaluated. Generally, managers, practitioners and citizens go about their business as if evaluation and reports do not exist.

The purpose of evaluation is to enable evaluation users to make better informed decisions and actions, thus the better to achieve what is important to them. Evaluation adds to the information that people have and improves the way they judge value, so that they can make more informed decisions than they would otherwise do.

How evaluation does this is to clarify the criteria used in the evaluation for judging value, so that people can decide whether or not to accept these criteria or how much weight to give them in making their own value judgement. It helps decisions by giving information about the intervention and its performance in relation to these criteria. But people will decide how to act by using criteria and values not included in the evaluation, and also by making judgements about the feasibility and consequences of different actions.

. . . or understanding causal mechanisms and generalizable principles . . .

This last part of the definition draws attention to the fact that the primary purpose of some evaluations is only scientific knowledge, and here evaluation clearly overlaps with more fundamental scientific research. Medical researchers and other scientists use certain evaluation designs because they are useful for investigating cause–effect mechanisms in different phenomena and for explaining and predicting. The 'general principles' refer to the aim of most evaluations being to produce findings which can be generalized beyond the specific intervention studied, thus this makes evaluation more than consultancy or development work.

Summary: what are the basic ideas?

- *Intervention: the thing being evaluated*: What is done to change what otherwise would have happened (*inter-venire*).
- *Implementation*: Actions and methods (strategy), people or groups doing the implementation and their connections (structure), systems such as those for data gathering and reporting, and support such as an innovative or culture which is ready to change.
- *Helpful and hindering factors*: What helps and hinders the take-up of the intervention/change in the immediate and wider environments?
- *Outcomes*: What 'comes out' of the intervention?
- *The difference the intervention makes*: Many results, both short- and long-term.
- *How do we collect data about outcomes?* Before/after indicators or measures; informants' views about what the results were.
- *Criteria and stakeholders*: Stakeholders: those who think they gain or lose from the intervention.
- *Criteria*: What is important to them about the intervention – what they value.
- *Attribution*: What caused the outcome? How do we know the outcomes were due to the intervention and not to something else?
- *Confounders*: Other things which could explain the outcome. These 'confuse' our understanding of the results of the intervention.
- *Controls*: What we do to control the influence of confounders.
- *Design*: What type of comparison is used, the times and methods for data collection, best presented in a diagram with a time-line.
- *Generalization*: Can the intervention be implemented elsewhere, under what circumstances? Would others find similar results to those reported in the evaluation if the intervention were implemented as in the evaluation (reproduced with fidelity)?

Approaches to evaluation

There are many designs and methods used in evaluation. The key to a good evaluation is to choose the design and methods which are most suited to the users' questions and to the type of intervention or change, but to do so within the constraints of time and resources for the evaluation.

Later chapters say more about designs, how to modify them and about how to get the best match between design and users' needs, within the constraints. The designs are grouped into three evaluation approaches:

1 *Experimental and quasi-experimental*: the intervention is treated as if it were an experiment and usually planned ahead, with data collected before the intervention are introduced, and then at a later time.
2 *Observational and naturalistic*: the evaluator observes the intervention in its natural setting and collects data about it to describe it and its effects. Sometimes also to evaluate how it was implemented in the study setting.
3 *Action evaluation*: feeds back data to implementers to improve the intervention and its implementation, sometimes to change these during the implementation. This may use any of the designs in the two groups above, but more often uses observational designs.

Assumptions about the intervention and the evaluation about the subjects to be changed

Every evaluation carries with it a conception of the subject which the intervention is seeking to change. A drug treatment for an individual can be assessed as an intervention to a biophysical system which operates according to natural laws outside of human consciousness. Or it can be assessed in a way that includes the patient's perceptions possibly influencing these processes, and their perceptions also will be an important outcome. As human beings, we function according to natural biophysical processes, but we also function according to how we understand ourselves and others, and these understandings affect our natural biophysical processes as well as our behaviour.

One point is that both interventions and evaluations involve assumptions about the subjects of the intervention: is the intervention to a machine or biological process, or to a conscious human subject, or to a work organization which operates in a different way from an individual? And for interventions to populations or communities, the intervention and the evaluation already have assumptions about this type of subject. Is it a collection of individuals with no relationships between them, or a social group with specific connections which affect how they respond to the intervention? A second point is that evaluators often make assumptions about the intervention regarding the nature of the subject that the intervention is intended to change. For example, concentrating on measuring biological outcomes and not measuring patient perceptions. Or measuring the effects of training without measuring any changes to culture or working arrangements. Evaluators need to be aware of these assumptions as an understanding of these is important to explaining the outcomes observed.

These differences in type of subject and assumptions about them are the reason why the chapters in Part II are divided into evaluations of interventions to patients, to individual providers, to service organizations, to health systems and to populations or communities. More on this later.

Match the evaluation design and criteria to the evaluation users' needs

A final note on users' needs and value criteria, as these are so central to carrying out an effective evaluation. Evaluations assess whether the change was effective according to one value criteria or more. This book proposes that they are best designed to meet the needs of a particular user: that they are planned and carried out for a particular user-customer.

There are two main groups of evaluation user. The first are patients, or practitioners who need the evaluation to help to decide what to do, such as clinical professionals, managers, purchasers, regulators or policy-makers. The second are researchers or academics, who often set their own criteria for judging the value of the intervention evaluated, which may or may not coincide with those of others.

Each group has different criteria for valuing the effectiveness of an intervention. The danger is trying to satisfy them all, which results in an inconclusive and superficial evaluation which is of little use to anybody. In later chapters, we consider how to address the challenges of defining users' value criteria and their decisions which the evaluation is to inform.

Evaluation for action does the following:

- recognizes the different perspectives of different groups ('stakeholders') who have an interest in the results of the evaluation and in the item being evaluated (it is politically aware);
- uses criteria agreed by one or more stakeholder groups (the primary users of the evaluation) to decide which data to gather and how to judge the value of the item (it is criterion-based);
- considers, at each step of the evaluation, the practical actions which the findings imply and which others might take if they were to act on the findings (action orientation is an integral part of the approach);
- uses the most relevant theory and methods from different disciplines for the purposes of the evaluation, to help decide the evaluation criteria, to gather and analyse data, and to clarify the implications for judging value and for carrying out action (it is multidisciplinary);
- covers the phases of defining the item to be evaluated, clarifying the evaluation criteria, gathering and analysing data, and judging value and planning and carrying out action.

Does this mean that the purpose of evaluation is change per se? Certainly, to change what users would otherwise have done: the aim is to enable practitioners, managers and others to do things differently and better as a result of the evaluation. The aim of evaluation, like the aim of a health intervention, is to make a difference. Even if the difference is only that people continue to do what they did before, but with more confidence that they are doing the right thing.

Action evaluations often will contribute to improving the change while it is being made. But how can you evaluate something while you are changing it at the same time? Here we touch on one of the differences between various evaluation perspectives: usually evaluations using an experimental perspective do everything they can to ensure that the intervention does not change during the evaluation. Action and developmental evaluations often feedback findings to people in a service during the evaluation so that they can make immediate changes.

The main point here is that the purpose of evaluation is practical action. 'Evaluation for action' is thus a broad umbrella term for a variety of different approaches which can be used for the purposes of practical improvement. It extends beyond the phases of an evaluation study which are usually described in research-oriented evaluation texts because evaluation for action pays attention to how to assist the practical actions which could follow from the data gathering.

Seven common shortcomings of evaluations

1. *Not describing the intervention actions*: How do we know what was evaluated? Could we repeat it from the description?
2. *Not describing the conditions under which the intervention or change was made*: How can others reproduce the intervention, especially if these conditions are necessary for implementation?
3. *Not defining the evaluation user and their value criteria*: How do we know what is important to users for them to act?
4. *Gathering data on too many outcomes*: Better to gather fewer data that are valid than a lot of data that are questionable.
5. *Gathering not enough data on outcomes*: Especially about possible negative results or long-term results.
6. *Assuming only the intervention could cause the outcome*: Not assessing other possible influences.
7. *Not considering the resources the intervention requires*: Not necessarily through a full economic evaluation, but at least noting the resource implications of the evaluation findings.

Conclusion

If evaluation were a religion, this would be a popular liberal Buddhist text on evaluation. This does not mean that it views life as suffering, though evaluations often do so because evaluators are usually someone's enemy. Neither is its aim peace or ultimate enlightenment, though a little of the latter may come. Compassion helps too. Rather, it is because it gives a plural and pragmatic approach: an experimental evaluation may be better than an observational design – it all depends on the user and their needs. There are certain tried and tested principles, but there is no one way. The evaluator and user must choose what is likely to work by looking at examples and others' experience.

As the result of an evaluation, someone should be better able to act or make a decision. This is more likely if the evaluation is designed with the user, using their criterion of valuation and to provide them with actionable information. Like an intervention, the evaluation should 'come between' what would otherwise have happened – it should make a significant difference to the user to be worth the time and cost.

The following chapters discuss the principles and concepts, and the eight steps in carrying out an evaluation. Part II shows designs in action in different example evaluations. Part III gives guidance on special subjects, including evaluating implementation, return on investment, and digital technologies.

2 Evaluation tools and concepts

Introduction

The idea of an 'intervention', or the change to be evaluated, is the single most important idea in this book. What was done differently which was not done before, such as a treatment or computer support or visits from expert health volunteers? Can we know what the outcomes are, or if it makes a difference if we do not know what the 'it' is which we are evaluating? Do all evaluations give a good description of the 'it' or 'the intervention' which they evaluate, which allows others to copy it if it works?

The idea of 'an intervention' or what was done differently is a 'tool for thinking'. Other 'tools for thinking' or concepts which we need to understand or carry out an evaluation are the subject of this chapter, such as the evaluation 'user', who is the customer of the evaluation.

After reading this chapter, you will be able:

- to quickly understand an evaluation you read and its implications by using ten concepts to analyse it;
- to speak the language of evaluation, which is based on these ten concepts, and be able to discuss evaluations with others;
- to quickly see the strengths and limitations of a particular evaluation, and use evaluation concepts to design your own evaluation.

An example evaluation

Concepts need examples to be understood. In this chapter, we will use the example evaluation below to illustrate what the concepts mean. We will revisit this throughout the chapter. What is 'the intervention' evaluated in this example?

Example: Is active multidisciplinary rehabilitation more effective than traditional primary care rehabilitation?

An active multidisciplinary rehabilitation programme provided by an occupational health unit was compared to a traditional primary care rehabilitation service in one area of Sweden. The patient groups compared were working people with neck or shoulder disorders who consulted physicians in each service over a three-month period. Patients were selected for both groups if they had not been on continuous sick leave for the disorder for more than four weeks before, or did not have other serious health problems.

One group received eight weeks of active multidisciplinary rehabilitation which involved physical training, education, social interaction and workplace visits. The primary care control group were given physiotherapy, medication, and rest or sick leave, as thought necessary by the physician.

The outcomes measured in both groups were the average number of days of sick leave for two years after the rehabilitation. Self-reports of symptoms and pain on a questionnaire were gathered before and at 12 months and 24 months. A short version of the sickness impact profile was used before and at 12 months to measure health-related behaviour such as mobility, social behaviour and recreational pastimes. Also at 12 months after the rehabilitation, patients were asked about changes in the workplace.

The findings were that there was no significant difference in outcome between the two groups. However, changes in the workplace such as new tasks or a new workplace were associated with decreased sick leave. This effect was found for both groups and was independent of the type of rehabilitation programme which they received.

(Ekberg et al. 1994)

Applying the tools

Do you already know how to use some of the tools?

- What was 'the intervention' in the example: an occupational health unit, or a traditional primary care rehabilitation service, or a physician consultation, or an active multidisciplinary rehabilitation?
- How were the outcomes measured?
- Were there controls, so as to help assess how much the intervention and not something else caused what the study says were the outcome differences?
- What were the value criteria used to assess the value of the intervention, and were the measures a valid way to obtain data about these value criteria?
- Who were the users of the evaluation?

Evaluation concepts discussed in this chapter

The chapter will now describe ten evaluation concepts and demonstrate why they are tools for thinking, to plan and use an evaluation properly:

1 *The user*: the people for whom the evaluation was designed, to help them make a more informed decision, e.g. a patient taking a drug to reduce blood pressure.

2 *Value criteria*: what is important to the user of the evaluation, for their decision or action, e.g. a drug to reduce blood pressure has few side effects and they will live longer because they take it.
3 *The intervention*: the thing or action being evaluated. What is done to try to change 'what otherwise would have happened' (*inter-venire*), e.g. a drug to reduce blood pressure, or, more broadly, a drug plus reminders and assistance to keep taking it properly.
4 *The implementation*: the actions taken to enable people to 'take up' the intervention, or introduce it into their daily practice or lifestyle or establish it in a community, e.g. help of different types to enable a patient to acquire the drug and keep taking it properly. (Sometimes implementation is not separated from the intervention, and is viewed as part of the intervention.)
5 *The critical environment conditions*: what helps or hinders applying the intervention and its operation in practice, e.g. the cost of the drug to the patient, friends and media who say it is not worth taking, a celebrity who says they are only alive because they take the drug.
6 *The subjects, intervention participant or 'target'*: the person, population, organization, process or thing to be changed by the intervention, e.g. the patient taking the drug.
7 *The outcome: any consequences or results of the intervention*: what 'comes out' of the action taken, e.g. ideally lower blood pressure (intermediate effect) and lower mortality (end result), but also less money to spend on other things because of the cost of the drug, plus a nearly infinite number of other outcomes including undesired side effects.
8 *The objectives (of the intervention/change)*: various, but usually the difference which the intervention is intended to make to (or with) the subjects. The intended outcomes for the subjects (the 'target' people), e.g. lower blood pressure.
9 *The confounder*: what confuses or can 'mix with' the intervention or the subjects, so that we cannot be confident if it was the intervention or something else which caused the outcomes, e.g. the patient suddenly gets serious about changing to a 'low blood pressure diet' and does not tell the evaluators.
10 *Control*: what is done to hold confounders constant, or to exclude them from having an influence, e.g. other patients do not get the intervention, but are equally likely to experience confounders, and outcomes are measured for them; or statistical calculations after data gathering, to check if patients in the two groups are different in a way which is significant.

Concept 1 The evaluation 'user' or 'customer'

Who uses an evaluation and why? Should evaluations be designed for just one user-group?

Users are the people for whom the evaluation was designed, to help them make a more informed decision. Examples of users of evaluations are health professionals, managers, patients, policy-makers such as politicians and their advisors, and those paying for healthcare (payers).

Who are the primary users of the example evaluation report about an 'active' and a 'traditional' rehabilitation programme above? Is it the managers, the professionals or others? A clue to deciding who the primary users are is to look at which measures were used and which data were collected. These include data about sick leave, about symptoms and pain, and about the impact on the sickness on health and lifestyle. Who is interested in these data and which decisions could these data help them to make? We can guess that the main users are professionals and managers and possibly payers and patients.

The main question is: who is the primary user? Many people read and use evaluation reports, but the 'users' are the people for whom the evaluation was designed. Managers and professionals will use an evaluation of a home care service for people returning home from hospital after surgery. But so will patients organizations who have particular concerns about the patients' experiences and how the services support the patient's carers. But the more users which an evaluation tries to serve, then the less well it serves any. The design becomes confused and there are not enough resources to collect all the different data which are required for the different interest groups. Many evaluations are inconclusive because they try to serve too many different users and different stakeholder perspectives. One reason that many evaluations are not acted on are that they are not designed for and with specific users, to take account of the information which they need for their decisions. This is why this book proposes a user-focused approach. Note that the primary user can be other researchers or the 'scientific community'.

The evaluator serves, but is not a servant of the user.

Concept 2 The value criteria

What is important to you as a patient if you are being treated for cancer or diabetes? Is it the same things that are important to an insurance company paying for the treatment being evaluated?

The value criteria are what is important to the user of the evaluation. Examples of criteria for judging the value of an intervention are: that it alleviates symptoms or cures, that a person lives longer, that the experience of undergoing a treatment is not painful, that a training programme is not boring, that there are no harmful side effects, that the amount of resources used by the intervention are not excessive, or how easy it is for people to carry out a treatment or reform.

What were the criteria which were used to judge the value of the rehabilitation treatment? Looking at the outcome measures, we would assume that the criteria of valuation were ability to work (as indicated by sick leave claims), reduction of pain, and return to previous activities and functions.

How did the evaluators decide these value criteria? Probably by thinking about what is important, but also about what was measurable in practice, and also by looking at what other researchers had measured. We do not know if they consulted users, but they may have imagined what would be important to them. Many research evaluations are oriented towards using the measures and value criteria which researchers have used previously. This may or may not be useful to practical users.

One danger is that the evaluator adopts too many criteria for valuing the intervention: the users' criteria, some from previous research, and their own, such as quality of life. This makes design and data collection almost impossible. The fewer the users and value criteria, the easier the evaluation. All evaluations are limited and partial. The question is whether the evaluation describes honestly, and proudly, these limitations and is self-critical.

Value, like beauty, is in the eye of the beholder, or user of the evaluation.

Concept 3 The intervention

The intervention is the thing or actions being evaluated. For 'things' other than a drug or a medical device, it can be difficult to define exactly what is and is not being evaluated. In the example, the intervention was an 'active multidisciplinary rehabilitation programme' and it was necessary to specify what to include in this and what to exclude. It is helpful to use the meaning of 'intervention' to work out exactly what are the boundaries of the intervention or whether in fact the boundaries may change (a subject we will return to later). Intervention comes from the Latin words 'inter' and 'venire' which mean 'between' and 'comes'. Or to put it another way, the intervention comes between 'what otherwise would have happened'. In one sense this is an inaccurate word to use for the thing we are evaluating, because the purpose of the evaluation is to see if the thing does make a difference: calling it an intervention assumes that it does. One way to think about it is to ask what was done differently and not done before, with the intention of making a difference. This is what we will evaluate.

To know what the intervention is, we must ask what is there now which was not there before. In the example, this was a 'multiple component' rehabilitation programme of physical training, education, social interaction and workplace visits. Examples of other interventions we evaluate are a treatment, or a chronic care treatment model, or training and feedback for clinicians, or a new payment system, or a set of activities to increase 'healthy ageing' in a population.

Concept 4 The implementation

What was done to establish this new rehabilitation programme described earlier? Actually, the report summary in the example does not describe how the rehabilitation programme was established – how the providers were recruited and trained and other actions taken to set it up so that it could be evaluated. Can we replicate the intervention, if it turns out to be very effective, if the implementation actions are not described? My view is, we might be able to, but we might save time if the evaluation described how the service was implemented or gave an appendix report on this.

> To define something is to decide the limits of it. It is not always easy to separate the boundary of an intervention from the actions taken to implement it or from its environment.

Tools for defining an intervention, action or change to be evaluated

Three features of an intervention or change are significant for the evaluator: the specifiability of the intervention, its stability, and its length of time. For example, a drug treatment is easy to describe and to specify the amount and how it is taken. This makes it possible to implement it consistently. It is stable (does not change), and we can describe the period of time over which it was taken.

Questions which help to define an intervention are:

- *Components?* These are the different parts or actions of an intervention. Both active rehabilitation and the primary care rehabilitation in the example had different components. Breaking down an intervention into its component parts helps to describe it.
- *Change?* This question is whether the intervention changes during the evaluation. Complex interventions, such as most health reforms, inevitably change over time. Does the report describe the change? How will an evaluator collect data about the change and how will they take this into account when they make their report? In the example, the report did not describe any significant change to the rehabilitation programmes during the period they were given to patients.
- *Boundary?* The third question is, where does the boundary lie between the intervention and its surroundings or 'environment'? The boundary separates the action which is evaluated from other things. It has to be clearly defined by saying what is and what is not the intervention. In the example, the rehabilitation programmes were separated from other things like a change to work-task or place of work.

A common shortcoming of evaluation reports is that they do not clearly describe the intervention or change which was evaluated. This makes it difficult for the reader to understand exactly what was evaluated, or to repeat the intervention and get the same results.

Concept 5 The critical environment conditions

The intervention is surrounded by an 'environment'. In the example, there are many features of the immediate and broader environment: it was in one area of Sweden with cultural norms regarding work, disability and using rehabilitation, within a broader environment of a welfare system which gave benefits for work disability. But which of these might influence the outcomes measured?

The evaluation is trying to find out how much the intervention caused any changes in the outcomes. That is, did it make a difference to these points?: number of days of sick leave; people's reports of symptoms and pain on a questionnaire; and health-related behaviour. But could other environment conditions be influencing these outcomes? Could a change to disability benefits influence the number of days a person takes off sick? Could the weather have an influence?

In this example, there was a control group who received the traditional intervention. The theory is that they were exposed to the same environmental influences as those receiving the intervention, which should mean any difference between the groups is only due to the intervention.

But what if there were no control group? In evaluations without control groups, it is necessary to consider the possible environment influences which could affect outcomes and to assess how much they might have done so. Even in evaluations with controls, it may be useful to collect data and describe environmental conditions because this influences how easy it is to implement the intervention, thus giving others a way of assessing what they might need to consider when they are implementing it.

The evaluation would not describe all the features of the environment, which is impossible anyway, just those features which may influence its implementation and outcomes. How do we know what these features are? We don't – we need to build a 'programme theory' to decide which data about the environment to collect. Chapter 9 shows the theory for a programme to reduce heart disease in a community.

Concept 6 The subjects, intervention participant or 'target'

Traditionally, the people, organization, or process to be changed by the intervention are called the 'target'. The people who were receiving the rehabilitation services were the targets in the rehabilitation example. I do not like using this word in this way – for two reasons. First 'target' can be confused with the aim or objective of the intervention, which is to have specific effects, such as reducing the time off work. Second, it implies that the people are passive recipients of the intervention. Yet for many interventions, patients or providers who are intentionally 'exposed' to an intervention choose whether or to be influenced by it and are not passive. They are subjects in the sense of being active agents. Similarly, 'implementation' is a poor word to describe whether and how patients or providers 'take up' an intervention.

'Subjects' is not the best word either, but it is better than 'intervention participant', which is more descriptive of the idea, and it will be the term used in this book. The book will sometimes use the word 'target participants' to describe those to be changed by the intervention when this is necessary.

Does the report describe characteristics of the subjects which may be important? For example, how long they had a neck or shoulder disorder before they received the intervention, or their age and sex? These characteristics may affect how the patients respond to the treatment, and knowing this helps the reader to judge if they would obtain similar results with their patients, or population or organization. Other data about the subjects are also needed, such as how many of the original group do not complete the treatment ('drop-outs') and why.

It is easy to describe and collect information about the subjects for most services, health programmes and training programmes. But the subjects of some health policies and health reforms are more difficult to describe. What is the subject (the target) of a decentralization reform? Is it the organizations at different levels of the health system? Subjects (targets) are always people, but sometimes it helps to think of an organization or a process as a subject, especially when evaluating a change to an organization or a new financing method. The main question is, who or what does the intervention aim to change? For a health reform, it may be necessary to separate immediate subjects (e.g. health professionals) from ultimate subjects (e.g. patients or the population).

An intervention does not just affect the subjects. The example evaluation only collected data about the subject patients. It did not collect data about how carers, employers or health providers were affected by the programme – the difference it made to them. The next section distinguishes the outcomes for the targets from the outcomes for other people.

Concept 7 The outcome

The outcome of an intervention is what 'comes out of it': the results or consequences. It is the difference which the intervention makes for the subjects, but also for other people. The measured outcomes reported in the rehabilitation example are sick leave, pain symptoms and activities and functions for the patients. The example does not report the effects of either programme on family members, health personnel, work colleagues or employers. Neither does it report how many resources are used, which is one outcome described in economic evaluation studies.

Most evaluations concentrate on finding out if the intervention does have the effect which is predicted or expected. They find what they are looking for but do not look for what they don't expect or don't want to find. There may be both unintended and undesirable outcomes to an intervention. We are learning from evaluations of some digital health technologies that they can result in harm to patients when we include data-gathering to check for such outcomes. Note also that outcomes do not always have to be measured numerically. Outcomes are not always numbers but can be people's perceptions which are then represented in an evaluation as quotes or as categories of types of perception such as 'difficulty in using the device'. This is why the book refers to outcome data rather than outcome measures as data can be qualitative or quantitative.

All interventions have 'side effects'. Some evaluations gather data to check for possible side effects, but few gather enough data to discover unpredictable or unexpected outcomes, especially those which only appear over the longer term, such as the need to replace an artificial hip six years after the hip replacement. The 'scope' of the outcome data refers to how broadly the evaluators look for different types of outcome – not just those which are intended for the subjects (targets). 'Scope' refers to how 'wide' the evaluation data-gathering 'net' is 'thrown' and the timescale over which the data are collected. A wide scope will be more likely to capture unintended outcomes but is more expensive and takes longer.

Outcomes: types and scope

Table 2.1 Example outcomes of a drug treatment

	Short-term	Long-term
Subject's outcome		
Intended (predicted?)	Symptom relief	Return to work
Unintended: good	Lower blood pressure	Sustained
Unintended: bad	Nausea	Dependence
Other outcomes (not for the subjects)		
Intended (predicted?)	Time and money consumed	Money saved
Unintended: good	Simpler to administer	More savings
Unintended: bad	Supplier raises prices	Personnel misuse the drug

Concept 8 The objectives (of the intervention/change)

One way to evaluate something is to assess to what extent it achieved its objectives. Did the rehabilitation programme in the example achieve the objectives set for it, regardless of other things? This depends on having a clear statement of the objectives of a service, programme, policy or reform. No objectives were stated for the programme in the evaluation report, but we could imagine that the objectives were related to the criteria of valuation: ability to work, pain relief and return to function.

In my experience, it is unusual to have clear and evaluable statements of the objectives of an intervention. For example, one service had as one of its objectives: 'Our objective is to give physiotherapy as soon as possible after referral by the physician.' This statement does have a general aim, but it is not a specific and measurable objective in the sense defined here. It is an action, not an objective: it does not define the target people (the subjects of the intervention) or an intended outcome for them (how they should be different) or any specifics about how they should be different. An objective is an intended outcome for the subjects, for example, that 'after five sessions of physiotherapy patients should report 50 per cent less back pain and 30 per cent return to function as defined by the function measure.' One way clearly to define an objective is the measurable difference the intervention is intended to make to the subjects and by when.

Having said this, I need to be fair to busy practitioners. Sometimes it is easier to define objectives in terms of activities, not in terms of what we want to achieve as results. Stating activities is a good first step towards defining objectives because we can then think about what difference our activities will make for the subjects (targets) of the activities. One way to do this is to ask, 'Why'? Ask, 'Why do we want to give five sessions of physiotherapy as soon as possible after referral?' And keep asking 'Why?' to become more specific.

Evaluators often have to take badly defined aims or objectives and define them in a way in which they can be evaluated. This may involve working with service providers to construct a definition of the objectives of the intervention. The concepts below help to write better objectives:

Intervention>>> Outcome for the subjects>>>Measure of outcome for the subjects

(ACTION) (RESULT) (INDICATOR)

Evaluators usually have to separate lower and higher objectives (e.g. objectives from higher aims), then separate actions from results, and then decide which measures/ data to collect on the results.

Concept 9 The confounder

Confounders are things other than the intervention which might cause the results. They are certain features of environment which are helpful or hindering influences. Confounders are what confuses or what 'mixes with' the intervention or the subjects so that we cannot be confident if it was the intervention or something else that caused the outcomes. In the example, the enthusiasm of the personnel to show that the programme was effective could have 'mixed with' the rehabilitation programme. So could patients feeling that they were getting a special service, and possibly patients being treated differently by their employers because they were in the programme. All are possible confounders.

All evaluations have to wrestle with the problem of 'attribution'. This is, how do we know that the intervention caused the result, and not something else? We can never be certain, but we have to consider other explanations and their plausible influence on outcomes, or assess the amount which these other influences may have contributed to any differences in before/after outcomes. When reading an evaluation we should imagine all the other things which could explain the results, apart from the intervention, and then judge whether the evaluators took these into consideration.

Designing out confounders

One way to exclude confounders is through designing the evaluation to do so. An example is to have two similar groups of people, and one group does not receive the intervention but is similar in all other respects to the group that does. Another way is to ask informants for their judgement on what 'came out' of an intervention. Then to ask them what else could also explain those outcomes, and ask them to assess how much these other things could have accounted for the outcomes.

Some evaluations not only try to find out if the intervention made a difference (outcome evaluation), but also how it worked. They try to identify the causal mechanisms and the factors which are essential for the intervention to have an effect – this is the 'programme theory' or theory of how the intervention worked to get the results. For example, how do the different components of the rehabilitation programme work to produce the outcomes? What is the pathway of influence which may lead to the final outcomes? Which environmental conditions are necessary for the programme to operate? Knowing this helps evaluation users to decide if they can replicate both the intervention and the results.

Concept 10 Control

Control is what evaluators do to hold confounders constant or to exclude them from having a possible influence. In the example, the evaluators used an intervention group of patients and a control group. The idea was to try to exclude such things as changes in the local area and other factors which could affect the outcome by comparing two groups where the difference was only that one group received the intervention and the other group did not. This is a common way to introduce control, as is also comparing one area or organization which was subjected to a change with another similar one which was not.

Is it possible to control all confounders? Practically, no. But also because we often do not know which factors and characteristics could also have an influence. What we can do is to try to increase our confidence that only the intervention caused the outcomes, and that the probability of the outcomes are greater than chance. Randomization of subjects goes a long way towards excluding such unknown factors, but this may not be possible, as we will see in the coming chapters. Often health programme or reform evaluations are not able to control confounders, and instead they seek to understand which factors affect the performance of the intervention – this is discussed in later chapters.

Discussion: separating intervention from implementation and environment

Why do we need to do this? Why do we need to distinguish between the intervention and the way it was put into practice or 'taken up' (implementation), and the environment within which it was taken up (e.g. the patient's biophysiology and social environment, the provider's peer group and culture, the organization's regulatory and financial environment, the community's wealth, culture and diversity)? We might not need to. As always, it depends on the user's question and need for information. If the user simply wants to know if it works in one respect, e.g. does it reduce costs in this one situation, then 'splitting hairs' like this may not be necessary. That is, so long as the evaluator includes the 'generalization disclaimer' in their report that 'these results might not be found elsewhere', it will be fine. But this limits the use of the evaluation to others, and may damage its publication value for those scientific journals that consider the main purpose of scientific research being to establish general principles or laws.

The point is to be aware of these distinctions for what we are evaluating and at least briefly consider what we would define as the intervention, its implementation and the environment. For some types of evaluation such as naturalistic evaluations of uncontrolled interventions, the distinctions are essential: the evaluator will need to spend some time separating these items in what they are studying.

To illustrate the distinctions between these elements, and why it is important to separate them, imagine that you are in hospital and you are unlucky enough to have a tube put in to take away your urine – a urinary catheter. The longer this tube stays in, then the more likely you are to get an infection. But nurses and doctors may be slow in taking it out when it is no longer essential. There are four steps to taking it out: (1) the physician recognizes it is in place; (2) they recognize it is no longer necessary; (3) they write an order to remove it; and (4) a nurse removes it.

The urinary catheter is an intervention to the patient. But here we will consider interventions to doctors and nurses, so as to get prompt removal of the catheter when it is no longer necessary. This is an improvement proved to be effective elsewhere in reducing infections. These interventions are of two main types: 'reminders' to remove; and 'stop orders' which are evidence-based prompts to physicians or nurses to remove it, for example, a day after surgery. Those are the interventions to providers.

But how are these interventions implemented? There are many ways to 'deliver' the intervention – to help the intervention be taken up. One is to have a one-day after surgery printed checklist which states to take it out if it is no longer necessary. Another is to have a computer-generated reminder or stop order. The point is that some evaluators looking at this topic distinguish between the intervention to providers – the reminders or stop orders – and the many different ways this intervention can be delivered – computer reminders, or verbal orders, or a printed checklist or a combination of them all.

Should the evaluator consider the environment within which this intervention is implemented? It depends on the purpose of the evaluation. Generally, for others to judge whether to use an intervention found effective in one place, then knowing both how it was implemented and the environment is important. For example, Janzen et al. (2013) used a combination of simple actions to speed appropriate catheter removal: (1) education for physicians; (2) a procedure requiring daily review; (3) posters; and (4) nurses encouraged to remind physicians to remove. There was a significant decrease in infections and length of stay. The environment factor arises when we ask, would others get the same results? The daily review was a simple add-on to the tasks in the daily routine face-to-face communication with the checklist at the bedside between the physician and nurse which was part of the local environment.

This 'environmental feature' is not the same in all hospitals. The fact that this add-on could easily be made a part of the already existing environment was important to its take-up and success. Other places might not have the same arrangements for communications and orders between nurse and doctor. So, describing the features of the environment which helped uptake was essential if others are to decide whether and how to implement the intervention.

Evaluation models or frameworks

A model which helps us to think about which data to collect for some types of evaluation is the Needs-Input-Process-Output-Outcome model (the NIPOO model) (Figure 2.1). This can also be used as the basis for a programme theory or logic model of the intervention in evaluations where it is useful to have one.

For health services or programmes, 'needs' refers to the health needs of the people who receive the intervention. In the rehabilitation service example, subjects are people suffering from neck and shoulder disorders and their main health needs are for cure or symptom relief. The inputs refers to all that 'goes into' the intervention. The evaluation will select which inputs to describe according to the evaluation user's needs for information. This may include a description of the intervention resources (e.g. the number and type of personnel working in the programme and the amount of time they give) and of the subject (e.g. the number and characteristics of the patients). In our rehabilitation example earlier, there was no description of resources for either programme, but there was a description of 'input' patient characteristics.

The 'process' is how the intervention is carried out and describes the different components, activities and procedures performed. There was little description of the process of either the active or traditional rehabilitation in the example evaluation report. Implementation is how the process is established: what is done to enable people to do the things which are described by the process. This was not described in the example either.

'Outputs' are the immediate products of the process, and are often described in terms of the number of patients who complete the process: in our example, we do not know how many patients finished each programme, only the numbers at two years for the follow-up data collection. 'Outcomes' are the difference the programme makes to the subjects such as patients, and to others, both short- and long-term differences. In the example, differences were measured before and at two years for sick leave, pain and mobility and functioning for the patients. No other outcomes were measured or reported.

The NIPOO model also demonstrates how some common value criteria can be measured. Efficiency is the ratio of inputs to outputs for one programme compared to another. For example, if the resource inputs for treating 50 patients with the active rehabilitation is costed at $25,000, then the cost per patient is $500. Efficiency is only really meaningful when compared with another programme, so we would also

Environment

Needs > Inputs > Processes > Outputs > Outcomes (short-term and long-term)

Targets________________ For subjects____________

For others____________

Figure 2.1 The NIPOO model

calculate the input–output ratio for the traditional programme. This may turn out to be $350 per patient, which would make the traditional programme more efficient.

But is the traditional programme more effective? In the rehabilitation example, we compare measures before and after to find the outcomes, and we discover that the outcomes are similar for the active and traditional programmes. Here we are defining effectiveness as whether the programme meets the health needs of people for whom it is intended. To describe effectiveness, we compare the health needs of people before with their needs after. Note, however, that there are other ways of defining efficiency and effectiveness – effectiveness is sometimes viewed as whether the programme met its objectives, even if meeting needs was not an objective.

Summary: how to do a useful evaluation

- Decide who the evaluation is for and what decisions it is to inform.
- Describe the intervention actions. (How do we know what was evaluated? Could we repeat it from the description?)
- Decide the conditions under which it was done.
- Don't gather too many outcomes data (better to gather fewer data that are valid than many data that are questionable).
- Don't gather too few outcome data (especially about possible negative results or long-term results).
- Don't assume only the intervention could cause the outcome. (Do not forget to assess other possible influences.)

Conclusion

The 'thinking tools', i.e. the concepts in this chapter help us to understand an evaluation and to see its limitations. They are also essential when designing an evaluation and are the basis for much of the discussion in the rest of this book as well as when discussing evaluations with others.

Evaluations are made to help people make better-informed decisions. To do this, evaluators need to know what is important to users for their decisions – the user's value criteria. The more users an evaluation tries to serve, then the less well it serves any. Many evaluations are inconclusive because they try to serve too many different users. A precondition for a good evaluation is to be able to limit it. Evaluators should aim to be reasonably certain about a few things. Perhaps the most common mistake made by evaluators is failing clearly to describe the intervention which they have evaluated.

3 Quick start

How do I plan and carry out an evaluation?

Introduction

If you want a quick 'how to' guide, this chapter presents eight steps for planning and carrying out an evaluation:

1 User goal specification
2 Reviewing relevant research
3 Defining practical and scientific questions
4 Listing and choosing designs
5 Preparing for the evaluation – practicalities
6 Data-gathering
7 Data analysis
8 Reporting, publishing and dissemination activities.

The chapter ends with the famous 'ADAGU' (**A**ims, **D**escription, **A**ttribution, **G**eneralization, and **U**sefulness) checklist: the five main questions to check your proposal or evaluation, and to assess others' evaluations.

Step 1 User goal specification

Who is the evaluation for and what should it enable them to do better? Answering this question defines the purpose of the evaluation, and from this, all else follows.

Key points

- Define the primary user group for the evaluation (the 'customer for the evaluation').
- Define the information they need to make their action or decision more effective – this is the difference they want the evaluation to make for them.
- Do this by working with users to agree the timescale and resources for the evaluation, and the type of information which different constraints will allow different evaluation designs to provide.

Who is it for and to inform which decisions?

If the single most important thing an evaluation has to do is to describe the intervention, then the single most important question it has to ask is, who is the evaluation for and to inform which decisions? All too often, evaluators or those paying do not start by answering this question. All else follows from this, and much wasted time and effort can be avoided by getting this right at the beginning of the evaluation.

In order to design the evaluation and data-gathering properly, the evaluator needs to be clear about who the evaluation is for (the user or customer of the evaluation), and the user decisions which the evaluation is intended to inform. The user's goals for the evaluation are the goals of the evaluator, e.g. 'I need to know if this intervention really does improve physicians' use of a clinical decision support, and by how much it does so.' Or 'I need to know if the strategy used by the service elsewhere is an effective way for us to implement a chronic care model.' This does not mean the evaluation cannot make suggestions – more on this later.

There are two types of user:

- a patient, or practitioner (clinician, manager or policy-maker);
- academic users (researchers and educationalists).

Researcher-evaluators are usually oriented to satisfying academics as their primary customer: other academics make decisions about funding or publications and this affects the researcher's academic career. But increasingly, funders, publishers and others are expecting an evaluation to have a direct practical use to practitioners. People are less willing to provide data or be involved if they cannot see the benefits. Funders sometimes do not use academics to review evaluation proposals. For some evaluations, funding is from service delivery budgets and the evaluation spends money which could be spent on other service operations. There are also evaluators outside of academia who are less bothered about publishing.

Evaluations that focus on one category of users are able to concentrate their resources, design and data-gathering on one purpose. No evaluation can answer all users' questions, and few can answer more than one or two. If performed well, there are usually publications which can follow, so long as the purpose and limitations are described in the publication.

Dialogue for defining the question and constraints

Specification of the users' goals for the evaluation is best carried out by the evaluator discussing and negotiating this with users or the funder. The evaluator needs to discover which decisions that the user needs to make which could be informed by the evaluation. Users will have many questions they want answered, but each extra question has a time and cost attached to it. Evaluators, like architects, need to show the different options and the costs and help the user think through what they most need from the evaluation. Researchers need to develop skills and methods to define, with the users, which primary questions are to be answered.

Even though this step is the most important, there are few methods and resources to help evaluators in this task, especially when working with users to define the question. Nearly all guidance is for academic research, which is primarily driven by previous research and disciplinary interests. It is certainly important to use previous research as part of the process of defining the question (see Step 2), but this should be only part of the process in a user-centred evaluation.

Defining who the user is may be easier than negotiating which of many questions the evaluation should answer. It also involves checking with the user whether an answer to these few questions can really make the user's actions more effective. Some general guidance about defining research questions is useful, especially the section on research questions given in Robson (1993). One short web resource is Apodaca (2013). For evaluations of some complex social interventions (CSIs), the five-step process by Preskill and Jones (2012) for engaging stakeholders in developing evaluation questions may be useful. This has four worksheets for a stakeholder 'engagement process'.

Craig et al. (2008) show, in their 'case study 14', an example of involving one type of user (a community) in the design and conduct of an evaluation. They propose that 'involving communities in the design of an evaluation is not just compatible with the use of rigorous methods, but can also improve them', and state:

> Memoranda of understanding were signed with community organisations to make explicit the obligations on both sides and the fact that all participants would receive the intervention. These organisations were closely involved in conducting the study, for example by organising community meetings in which the study was explained to possible participants, recruiting local interviewers, and organising meetings to disseminate early results. Local health workers were employed to recruit participants into the study.

Summary

An actionable evaluation does the following:

- is designed to give an evaluation 'user' or 'customer' evidence which helps them to make more informed decisions about what they should do, at the time when they need it;
- is best designed for one user, and uses their value criteria to decide which evidence to collect;
- states that many other outcomes are likely but were not investigated because of the limitations of the evaluation;
- involves collaboration with the evaluation user, to clarify why they want the evaluation, their questions about the intervention and outcomes, which decisions the evaluation is to inform, and which criteria to use to judge the value of the intervention;
- decides the design and data collection method to best meet the needs of the user within the timescale and resources available for the evaluation.

Does this mean that all evaluations concentrate on one group of users' questions and ignore the perceptions of the other stakeholders with an interest in a health programme or change? The answer is 'yes' – and 'no'. 'Yes', a focus on one group of users' questions and needs to inform decisions is necessary to deliver an evaluation which is more likely to be used to inform real decisions. The 'no' answer is that the evaluation does not ignore the perceptions which other groups have about the intervention or change, and does gather data from different perspectives. The reason is that, for the users to make informed decisions, they often need to know what different parties think about a intervention or change.

Step 2 Reviewing relevant research

Are the users' questions answered by already published research? Showing what is known and any gaps is necessary to avoid duplication and to obtain funding and be published.

Key points

- First, do a simple search with Google Scholar and then Pubmed. Set a time limit for this of two hours, and try different search terms.
- Depending on the time and resources available, do a more detailed search and keep a record of the search.
- Use the search findings in Step 3 to further define the evaluation question.

This step is particularly important if the primary users are other academics, and is also necessary for any publication in a peer-reviewed journal and to prepare a proposal for research funding: the purpose of academic research evaluations is to contribute to knowledge in the discipline. The review shows how the evaluation can do this and what is already known and where the gaps or controversies are in the literature.

Reviews can be simple, or long and complex, and everything in between. How much time is spent on this stage and which methods to use depend on the timescale and resources available. Rapid reviews are systematic, but are usually carried out with a six weeks to six months time target – one guide to such is Ganann et al. (2010). Mays et al. (2005) also give guidance on this topic.

Another method, where the literature is spread across many different databases, is to use a 'management review model'. This uses a database of published research, already completed evidence reviews, and the evaluator's existing knowledge of research on the subject in an iterative approach to combine different sources and types of evidence (Greenhalgh et al. 2004; Greenhalgh and Peacock 2005; Øvretveit 2012). The steps are as follows:

a *Broad scan.* Define the objectives and search terms for the review, find and note the literature on the subject.
b *Narrow the focus on previous reviews.* Identify and select previous reviews, assess these for answers to the review questions.
c *Open out inclusion.* Bring in high-quality individual studies in order to provide additional evidence to answer the review questions, noting the strength of evidence of the findings and assigning a grade score (e.g. the GRADE scoring system, see Guyatt et al. 2008).

d *Open inclusion more widely.* Add other research (of acceptable evidence strength) to fill in the evidence for the questions, noting that the evidence at this level is weaker, and using a snowball approach to identify relevant studies.
e *Review and synthesize.* Combine the evidence in order to answer the questions, noting the degree of certainty (through the grading system). Identify unanswered questions and priorities for research, and provide any recommendations that are supported by the evidence.

Step 3 Defining practical and scientific questions

The step brings the review of previous research together with the user definition of the purpose of the evaluation. This then helps to define both the practical and scientific questions to be answered by the evaluation.

Key points

- Define the evaluation parameters and resources: specify the report target date, the budget and skills available for the research, and how much data you can use which have already been collected.
- Be clear whether the primary users will be practitioners or the academic community.
- Define the practical questions as those which will ultimately reduce suffering and costs, and the academic questions as those which will build theory or contribute to the empirical knowledge which is shown to be needed by previous research. This then allows the choice of the design most suited to answering the questions within the constraints of time and resources available.

Step 4 Listing and choosing designs

Listing potential designs leads to a choice of which one will provide acceptable answers, within the timescale and resources available.

Key points

- The design is best presented in a time-line. It shows which data will be collected and when, and the comparisons to be made to answer the evaluation question.
- Some designs are automatically ruled out by the timescale and resources available for the evaluation, or by other constraints and practical issues.
- Experimental and quasi-experimental designs are suitable for questions on the effectiveness outcome.
- Observational designs can be used for both effectiveness and implementation questions.
- Action evaluations may be suitable for questions about how to improve the intervention while it is being implemented.

- When considering which outcome data to collect, consider whether accessible data already exist: any special primary data collection by evaluators is costly in time and money.

Some designs might not be feasible. For example, because comparison subjects are not available, or difficulties in randomizing units, or there were no time series data before the intervention was started.

The three most common types of comparison are:

- Between what was planned and which outcomes were achieved. (Did the intervention achieve the outcomes intended?)
- 'Before', compared to 'after' (or 'later'), referring to measures of a characteristic of the person or unit receiving the intervention. (Does this show the intervention made a difference in this characteristic?)
- Outcomes, compared to those of a comparison group (comparative effectiveness).

More details about each type of design are given in Chapter 4. The following references give the best overviews of different designs and their strengths and weaknesses: (Robson 1993; Øvretveit 1998, 2002; Tunis et al. 2003; Mercer et al. 2007; Craig et al. 2008; Fan et al. 2010).

There are different views about whether an evaluation framework or model of the intervention is part of the design stage, or part of 'preparing for an evaluation' (see Step 5). Such frameworks or models should certainly be considered in this, or the next step, as a framework helps to decide which data to collect and the methods to use.

Step 5 Preparing for the evaluation – practicalities

Preparation turns the design into who does what, and when, to find and analyse the data. Practical arrangements can be planned, using a time-task map. This also includes steps for ethical approval which is often necessary.

Key points

- Decide the date for the final activity in the evaluation (e.g. submission of report, or presentation to users).
- A simple Gantt chart lists the tasks in a vertical column, and the dates across the top row of the chart. Put this activity and date at the bottom of a Gantt chart (Figure 3.1). Start with the end in mind and work back from that date.
- List other activities and add them under the dates in the Gantt chart.
- Note any critical activities which need to be completed before the next set of activities can start.
- Note whether your earlier assumptions about the people, their skills and time for the evaluation still apply, and double-check their availability for the times suggested by the plan.
- List events which could slow down the evaluation and possible ways of predicting or mitigating these (i.e. risk management planning).

Timetable of the project

No.	Activity	Jan	Feb	Mar	Apr	Mar	Jun	Jul
		1 2 3 4 5	6 7 8 9	10 11 12 13 14	15 16 17 18	19 20 21 22	23 24 25 26 27	28 29
1	**Budgeting, contracting** -->15.Jan.2003							
	Project 15.Jan - 15.Jul							
2	**Introduction Meeting (Oslo)** 15.Jan - 17.Jan							
3	**Methodology** 15.Jan - 9.Feb							
4	**Background information** 15.Jan - 9.Feb							
5	**Interview planning** 17.Feb - 9.Mar							
6	**Coordin. meeting (Tallinn)** 10.Mar - 11.Mar							
7	**Fieldwork - interviews** 17.Mar - 6.Apr							
8	**Data writing out** 17.Mar - 13.Apr							
9	**Country data analysis** 24.Mar - 18.May							
10	**Country data translating** 19.May - 8.Jun							
11	**Half-way meeting (Oslo)** 11.Jun - 13.Jun							
12	**Data final analysis** 16.Jun - 6.Jul							
13	**Report writing** 16.Jun - 13.Jul							

Figure 3.1 A simple GANTT chart

Remember to reserve plenty of time to find out if approval from an ethics committee is required, and to apply swiftly if approval is needed. Some publications require proof that this has been done. If the evaluation aims to be generalizable, then it is called research, and in the USA this needs the approval of the local ethics Institutional Review Board (IRB). Some evaluations for quality improvement might not need IRB approval.

Step 6 Data-gathering

To answer the evaluation questions, data need to be gathered from different sources, using different methods and stored in a way to make analysis easy.

Key points

- Data can be in qualitative or quantitative form and collected using the data collection methods which are known to most researchers.
- Qualitative and quantitative data will be needed to describe the intervention which was actually implemented, and about possible outcomes at different times, as well as about the environmental conditions surrounding the intervention.

- Data about immediate and later outcomes are needed, which can be from quantitative before/after measures, or qualitative assessments about outcomes by informed observers.
- Which data to collect can be guided by a model or framework of the intervention, which shows the component parts of the intervention and different outcomes at different times.
- Try to use data that have already been collected which you can access, if these are of acceptable validity and reliability: any other data you collect yourself for the study will cost considerable time and money.
- Decide the best balance between concentrating resources on a few data collection methods to increase the reliability and validity of the data, and using a number of methods to see if the same findings are to be found in different data (i.e. data triangulation).

The ten golden rules for data collection

a Don't collect data unless you are sure no one else has done so already.
b Don't invent a new measure when a proven one will do. (Do we really need another quality of life measure?)
c When the person or documents you need to see are not there, don't be blind to what is there which could help – be opportunistic.
d Measure what is important, not what is easy to measure.
e Don't collect data where confounders will make interpretation impossible.
f Spend twice as much time on planning and designing the evaluation than you spend on data collection.
g Always do a small pilot to test the method on a small sample.
h As you collect the data, save them to a database which is designed with thought to how to carry out the analysis, and back it up every day! Expect all kinds of computer problems.
i Analysing the data takes twice as long as collecting it, if you have not defined clearly which data you need and why.
j Remember, data collection will always take twice as long as you expect.

Step 7 Data analysis

Use the data to describe the intervention or change which was actually implemented, the outcomes which are of interest and to note the limitations of the findings.

Key points

- Analysis is far easier and quicker if the data, when collected, were stored in a way which was organized with a view to how the data will later be analysed. So look ahead in Steps 4 and 5 to plan this.

- Analysis should start by describing the intervention or change which was actually implemented: what was implemented decides which outcomes are worth looking for in the data.
- Computer software for analysis of both quantitative and qualitative data can save time and money, but depends on using the software to explore questions defined earlier in the evaluation.
- If you are not familiar with the software, try to get an experienced researcher to guide you through how to use it on your data. Learn by doing: courses are expensive and many are not very useful.

Analysis starts by describing the complex social intervention (CSI) which was actually implemented. This is because some planned changes may not have been implemented. Therefore, some outcomes expected from these changes are not likely: time is better spent assessing outcomes which are likely from the changes that were actually implemented.

Step 8 Reporting, publishing and dissemination activities

An evaluation is only effective when it is used to decide what to do, such as whether or how to change a clinical intervention, a service or to make a change. The findings of the evaluation need to be communicated and be available to users at a time when they can use it to change what they would otherwise do.

Key points

- When writing, organize the evaluation report around users' questions: to be understood and used, evaluation reports need to be presented with headings and in a style that addresses these questions.
- Give a concise report, in a dispassionate style, presenting findings in visual displays with tables of numbers in appendices, and get the right balance between too many qualifications which make it difficult to read, and too few.
- Describe the limitations, so as not to mislead users who may see findings as being more certain than you know them to be.
- Give guidance on the conditions users would need to obtain similar results from implementing the intervention which was evaluated.
- There is a trend towards the evaluator's role extending beyond only sending a report, and towards advising users about implementation.

Evaluation alone changes nothing. For the evaluation to make a difference to patients or for costs, it needs to be available to decision-makers in a form and at a time when it will influence their actions at the 'window of action' time. Evaluators need to 'market' their report by identifying the users, discovering where users are likely to look for such information, and find ways to make summaries and the full report easily available.

The internet and databases which can be searched are important places where the report needs to be noted and be available. Some evaluations establish a website for the evaluation which is easily discovered in a search, allows downloading, and provides any supporting materials which can help evaluation users. Resources describing effective dissemination approaches are given by Research Utilization Support and Health (2009).

As regards the content of reports and publications, guides have been written about which information needs to be reported for different types of evaluation and audience, e.g. Boutron et al. (2008) (for randomized controlled trials, RCTs), and Ogrinc et al. (2008) (for quality improvement). The 'Reporting Guidelines 2013' list in the references in Ogrinc et al. (2008) gives more reporting standards guides. Most such guides emphasize describing details of the intervention and its implementation so that others can reproduce it. The detailed descriptions can be in a report appendix, or, for publications, in a web appendix, including assessments about what can and cannot be modified for the setting, patients or providers if similar results are to be expected.

Presenting some details of the setting for an intervention evaluated by a RCT is recommended in many reporting guides (Boutron et al. 2008). But for observational or action evaluations, such details of context need to be far greater. The need to report such descriptions shows the importance of pre-study planning and theory to decide which data to collect and how to collect them on the intervention and context during the evaluation. The later section of this guide describes frameworks for deciding which data to collect on context, which can also be used to decide how to present the information in the report.

All the above moves this guidance back to the first step of the evaluation. It shows the importance of identifying, right at the start, who the evaluation is for and which of their decisions are the focus of the evaluation.

Summary: how good is this evaluation for its purpose?

It is best when designing the evaluation to note the 'ADAGU' strategies which can be used in the evaluation to address each of these questions below. Stating these strategies will strengthen proposals for funding the evaluation, helps in developing innovations in design and makes the final report more useful. This is also a good checklist for quickly understanding an evaluation.

- **A**ims: what information is needed and what are the questions to be addressed?
- **D**escription: what are the details of the intervention, its implementation and context?
- **A**ttribution: how confident can we be that the intervention caused the outcomes reported?
- **G**eneralization: can we copy it and obtain similar results?
- **U**sefulness: in which situation are the intervention and implementation feasible and how do we enable users to use the findings from the evaluation?

Conclusion

No longer can evaluators expect patients or practitioners to give their data or time freely. User-centred evaluation focuses on the questions of one user-group, whether they are academics or those of patients or practitioners. This focus starts the evaluation with a chance of its being useful, and allows design and planning for a purpose. Start with the end in mind with Step 1 to clarify these questions, ideally in dialogue with users. Other chapters in this book provide more tools and guidance for each step.

4 Designs

Introduction

We need a design to depict the most important parts of the evaluation and to communicate this to others. Design illustrates which data will be collected and when, and shows the comparisons to be made to answer the evaluation question. Figure 4.1 gives an example of a before/after design.

This chapter gives an overview of the most common designs used by evaluators. The diagrams help to explain simply to people what the evaluation will do and when. You can find example evaluations of many of the designs in Part II of the book which says more about their strengths and limitations for different purposes. This chapter refers to these examples in Part II.

A design shows the logic of the evaluation, not the logistics which forms the more detailed practical timetabling for the evaluators and implementers of who does what, and when. The design does not show details of data collection methods, and the comparison can be simple, such as before and after the intervention – it does not always involve a comparison group.

Designs are best represented as a time-line, for example, Figure 4.2 shows time vertically, of an evaluation of an intervention by pharmacists visiting primary care centres to improve physicians' compliance with the guideline. This example is discussed in full in Chapter 6. The time-line starts at the top and goes down the page, and the outcome data to be collected are shown– the one thing that is missing is the times when these data will be collected. Part II discusses other types of picture to summarize different designs.

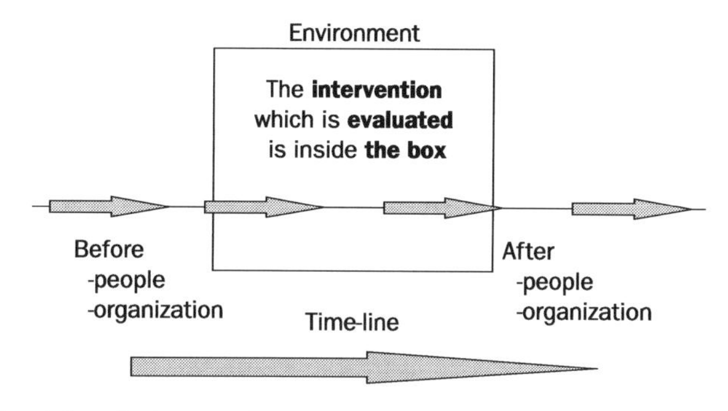

Figure 4.1 Before/after the intervention

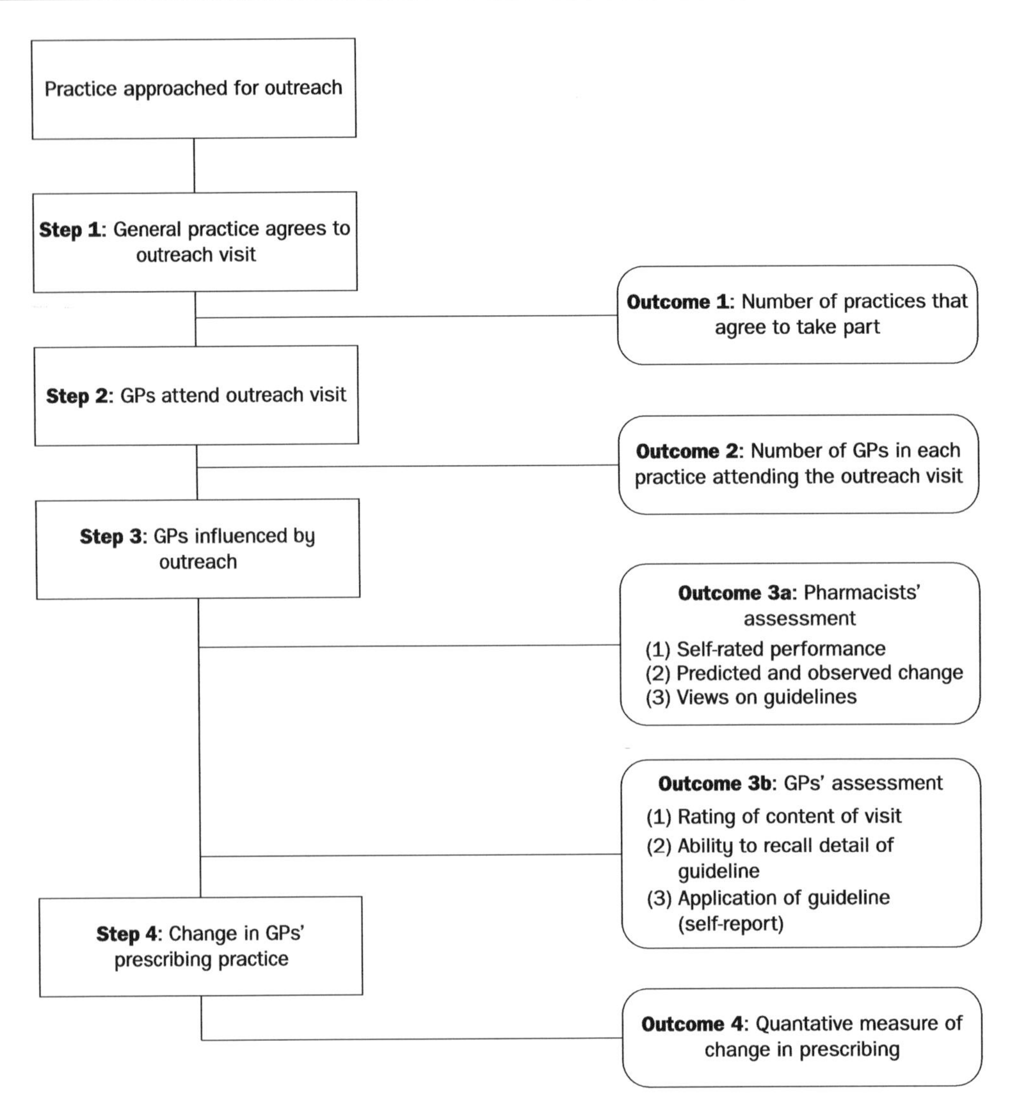

Figure 4.2 Pathway of change in general practitioners' (GPs') prescribing practice
Source: Nazareth et al. (2002),

Three types of design

The designs can broadly be divided into three types:

1 *Experimental and quasi-experimental*: In this family of designs, the treatment, change, service or programme evaluated is thought of as an experiment, and the change is planned before it is introduced. Data-gathering methods are piloted, and then 'baseline' data are collected before the intervention/change and again after

the intervention is introduced. Often the data are in quantitative form, from measures carefully selected to indicate any outcomes which are related to the evaluation user's questions and decisions. The summaries later start with the simpler single before/after quasi-experimental design, before then describing other designs which compare groups who receive the intervention to those who do not.

2 *Observational*: These designs are usually to evaluate interventions and changes in real-world settings and have fewer controls to rule out the explanations of outcomes other than the intervention. The fact that a pre-planned intervention experiment is not used does not mean that studies using this approach do not use other scientific techniques, such as formulating and testing hypotheses about the possible effects of the intervention or service on the subjects on which the data are gathered. This approach is used in many evaluations and termed 'formative', 'process', 'case', and 'programme' evaluation. Some designs in this category are called cohort, case-control and cross-sectional, usually if the data collected are quantitative in nature.
3 *Action*: The main difference from the other two approaches is that the evaluator does not try to minimize the effect of the evaluation on the intervention or service studied. Rather, the researcher-evaluator tries to help improve the service or intervention as it is implemented. Typically the researcher will present early findings to implementers, and sometimes help them to design and redesign the intervention (Øvretveit 1998, 2002).

The differences between experimental, observational and action evaluations are not the data collection methods they use: designs in all three can use data that are gathered quantitatively, or qualitatively or by mixed data collection methods. The differences are in the methods used to increase certainty that the outcomes are due to the intervention and not to something else.

Wagenaar and Komro (2011), referring to 'natural experiments' state: 'Combining many design elements into a single study can produce evaluations with high validity and strength of causal inference as good as, and sometimes better than, randomized trials.'

Experimental and quasi-experimental designs

Experimental designs are where the intervention is planned, as are the data to be collected. The intervention is then made as if it were an experiment: it is a forward-looking prospective design. This summary starts with the simpler 'quasi-experimental' designs.

Non-comparative quasi-experimental designs

Before/after design

The before stage is when the data are gathered. The after stage is after the intervention has been applied. Data are collected about a few features of the subjects to be exposed to the intervention before the intervention starts, such as blood pressure or prior knowledge. Then data are collected about the same features after the intervention to see if the intervention itself has changed these features. This is shown in Figure 4.1 on page 41. The evaluation comparison through which value is judged in this design is the before stage compared to the after stage.

The design involves listing other possible explanations for the before/after (or later) data differences and assessing their likely influence. But without a comparison group, these explanations cannot be excluded. People get better when they feel cared for, regardless of the medicine. A 'significant improvement' was reported in up to 40 per cent of patients with angina, severe post-operative pain, or cough when they were given assurance and a non-active pill (Beecher 1955; see also Benson and Epstein 1975 and Benson and McCallie 1979). While the effectiveness of 'tea and sympathy' and 'tender loving care' is well known to health workers, and these are recognized interventions, they do prove a problem for experimental evaluators who need to standardize the intervention.

A note by a famous experimenter, Benjamin Franklin, shows an early recognition of this problem. He wondered in a letter to a colleague whether the improvements in his patients were not in fact from the electric shocks he was giving them, but from 'the exercise in the patients' journey, and coming daily to my house, or from the spirits given by the hope of success, enabling them to exert more strengths in moving their limbs' (Franklin 1941). Thus, to find out if an intervention is effective, we do not compare it to nothing. One way of controlling for 'experimental effects' is to use one of the later comparison group designs, This involves a control group of subjects who get a 'placebo' intervention rather than nothing or, another treatment, as in comparative effectiveness research.

Time series design

This is like a 'before and after' design, but there are many before-data- and many after-data-collection time points for the outcome of interest. The idea is that a series of data points before show an average level over the period (e.g. data collected every month about infection rates for 12 months before any intervention). Then the intervention is introduced and the impact on the outcome data is assessed over the subsequent data points. If there is a significant rise, or none, each month after, for a period of time, then this gives an indication of the effect of the intervention. The time trends are also useful to see if any outcome is sustained. For example, one training event may show a sudden change to the outcome data but drop to the earlier levels after a few weeks. Figure 4.3 shows an example of a time series design.

The interrupted time series design is a variation on this: the intervention is introduced, and then stopped for a series of outcome data points, in order to assess whether the outcome data levels return to the average before. The interruption can be repeated, to increase certainty about whether the intervention really does affect the outcome. Example 3 in Part II uses this design.

If enough time data points are collected in the right way, then statistical process control (SPC) methods can be used to define upper and lower control limits and to

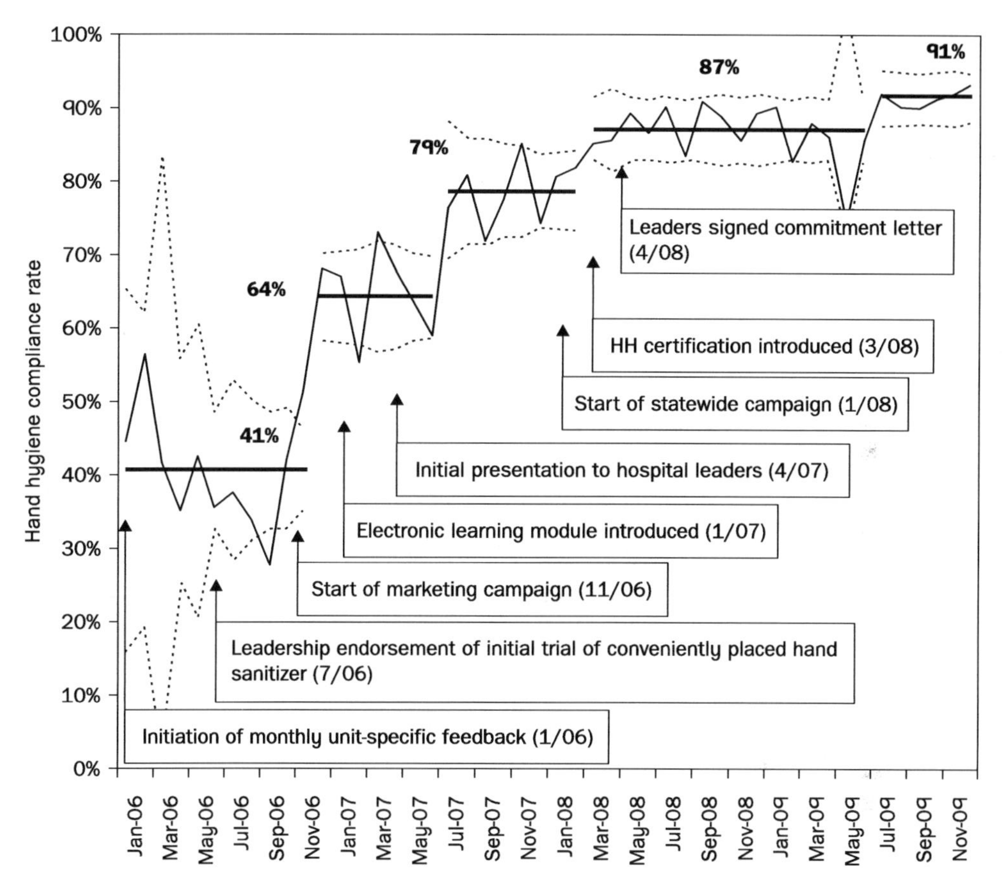

Figure 4.3 An example of a time series design
Source: Kirkland et al. (2012).

identify any special reasons (such as the intervention) that significantly change the process which are over and above the random variation which is to be expected (Wheeler 1993; Carey and Lloyd 1995).

Quality improvement testing (PDSA)

Many quality improvement interventions aim to change the provider behaviour, the care process or the organization. The plan–do–study–act cycle (PDSA) is an evaluation technique used in quality improvement to study whether a planned change, when implemented, has an effect on the outcomes of interest (Langley et al. 1996). If this testing cycle is applied with a certain rigour, and possibly also using a time series design, then some researchers view it as allowing a reasonable degree of certainty about the attribution of outcomes to the intervention in real-world settings, even without a control group. The design allows for, indeed requires, repeated changes to the intervention to check if revisions can improve the apparent impact on outcomes ('iteration testing' for 'continuous improvement'). In principle, some evaluations of this kind might also be classified as action evaluations where the evaluation is integral to intervention development and implementation.

The certainty of the attribution for evaluation can be enhanced by using the approach described by Speroff and O'Connor (2004): formation of a hypothesis for improvement (Plan), a study protocol with collection of data (Do), analysis and interpretation of the results (Study), and the iteration of what to do next (Act). Different designs can be used within this framework but the time series design, with or without statistical process control methods, is the most common.

Comparative experimental designs

Like the quasi-experimental designs these plan and implement a defined intervention-change to intervention subjects. The intervention could be for patients (e.g. a combination of services for patients with a chronic illness), or for providers (e.g. a combination of training and reminders to physicians to encourage compliance with clinical guidelines), or for service organizations (e.g. financial incentives and education to reduce hospital acquired infections) or a combination of interventions for patients, providers and service units.

The defining feature is that some subjects receive the intervention/change and some do not (the 'comparison' or 'control' group). Outcomes data are from measures which are selected to show the effects of the intervention. These data are collected before exposure ('baseline'), and then at one or more times after exposure, or 'later' if the intervention is sustained for some time.

Planning of, and controls in, implementation try to ensure each subject is 'exposed' to a standard intervention which is as similar as possible for all. The aim is to reduce possible variations between subjects in the 'dose' or 'frequency' of the intervention, so as to maximize the certainty of attribution to the intervention of any of the before/later differences in the outcome data which are documented by the evaluation. Having an evaluation protocol which describes the intervention clearly then can provide others with details of how to reproduce the intervention.

Randomized controlled trial (RCT)

A randomized controlled trial (RCT) is a comparative experimental design where the subjects are randomly allocated to be exposed to the intervention/change or some comparison intervention (or to none at all).

Randomization is important. The intervention is one of many things which may affect the outcome, for example, treatment outcomes are often different for men and women, smokers and non-smokers, or for older and younger people. In many patient groups there is a 'spontaneous improvement' over time. Random allocation with large-enough groups, and which has been preceded by careful selection, aims to ensure that the characteristics of people which could affect the outcome are evenly distributed between both groups, so that any outcome differences between the two groups can be attributed to the intervention.

There are many characteristics which we do not know about but which might affect the outcome – random allocation with enough subjects means that we can control for these as well. We use 'matching' of the subjects going into experimental and comparison groups when we cannot randomize – this is discussed later.

Why use statistics?

A key feature of experimental design is statistical analysis. You need statistics at the start to assess how many subjects to include in the trial. The reason is this: in RCTs usually a few measures are taken of each subject's physiology, health or behaviour or knowledge which the intervention is intended to change, which gives us numerical data of these features before and after the intervention.

Why would you need to work out how many subjects receive the intervention (the experimental group) and how many receive the comparison exposure which may be nothing (the control group)? Are you expecting a difference between these groups after the intervention? This design looks for a before/after difference for the intervention group in the same way that the simple before/after design does. But we have the control group to compare with as well. Might there be before/after differences in this group as well? Does comparing the size of the difference between the two groups help to see how much the intervention and not something else causes the difference?

The answer is 'yes' and 'no'. Yes, we can see if the subjects in the intervention group show a greater difference in the measured outcomes than those in the control group. But the size of this difference may not be significant. Even though we have a comparison group, if there is a small difference, for example, in mortality, or knowledge score in a test between the two groups, this could still be due to things other than the intervention. Randomization is intended to distribute subjects equally to the two groups with features which could cause them to respond differently. If we have 1000 subjects in the intervention group and 1000 in the control group, then these features would be nearly equally represented in both groups, and a small difference in the measures is likely to indicate the intervention effects. But if we only used ten subjects in both groups, then a small difference might be due to features of the subjects not the intervention.

So, why do we need statistics? The answer is that we guess how big the difference in outcomes measured might be between the intervention and control group subjects. Then, using statistics, we can estimate how many subjects we need for both groups to show a significant difference. If we expect the intervention to make a big difference, then we need fewer subjects because the size of the difference will be much larger than differences due to other causes. Then after the evaluation, we use statistics analysis to judge the significance of the results.

Another influence which could affect outcome is whether a person knows that he or she is in a control group or an experimental group. 'Single-blinding' is when the people in the control and the experimental group or site do not know which group they are in, but the people running the intervention do know. 'Double-blinding' is where both the subjects and the people running the intervention do not know which is the control group and which is the experimental group. 'Triple-blinding' is where even the evaluators do not know who is in which group until the experiment is over. 'Ethical blindness' is where evaluators do not tell subjects or care-givers that they are taking part in a pre-planned evaluation.

The important point is that randomization in sufficient numbers reduces the possibility of there being differences between characteristics of the 'intervention group' and the 'comparison group', which would make conclusions less certain about whether the outcomes were caused by the intervention rather than caused by a characteristic of the exposed subjects such as age or education. The example studies 1 and 2 in Part II illustrate how this design was used to evaluate two different interventions.

Features of an RCT design

1. Review of previous knowledge to specify the hypothesis to be tested.
2. Selection of subject people or sites for the test or trial.
3. An experimental and a control group (or site) of sufficient numbers.
4. Random allocation of subjects to each group.
5. A limited number of 'outcome' measures are made of the subjects in both groups which focus on effects (outcomes).
6. Statistical analysis to decide how many subjects (the 'power' of the trial) and to communicate the significance of the results (the confidence that the data difference is due to the intervention).

Glasziou et al. (2008) propose that RCTs are not necessary when the effect size is large, which, unfortunately, is rare for many interventions. Hawe et al. (2004) suggest that RCTs can be appropriate if a different approach to standardization is used:

> The issue is to allow the form to be adapted while standardizing the process and function ... For example, 'workshops for general practitioners' are better regarded as mechanisms to engage general practitioners in organisational change or train them in a particular skill. These mechanisms could then take on different forms according to local context, while achieving the same objective.

There is increasing criticism of the RCT design and some are noted in Part II. For now, two comments: first, most RCTs have traditionally not used subjective patient reports, but many more are now using such data-gathering methods. The criticism of a preference for some types of data-gathering method is not a valid criticism of the design principles. Second, if you had cancer and had to choose between different treatments, which evaluation would you look at first: one or a number of well-designed RCTs, or an evaluation of patients' subjective experience of the different treatments? There are not many things in life more certain than the findings of a meta-analysis of a number of high-quality RCTs which shows that the RCTs came to the same conclusions.

Non-randomized comparative trial

In this, subjects receiving the intervention and comparison subjects are 'matched' as far as possible for characteristics which might affect how they respond to the intervention. For example, if the patient is the unit in the intervention, the evaluators may try to assign patients to both groups who are similar in age, sex, education and income. However, the group receiving and not receiving the intervention may be different in other ways which are not matched but which can affect outcomes. These other characteristics add an influence other than the intervention and which confounds (confuses) the findings (Concato and Horwitz 2004; Concato et al. 2010). Just to confuse things, some writers classify a comparative trial as a 'cohort study' where the effects of an intervention on one 'cohort' are compared to the effects of an alternative or nothing on another 'cohort'. In this book, those designs like this which are not planned prospectively are called observational and are noted later.

Cross-over comparative trial

In this variation, one group receives the intervention, while the other group receives none or another intervention, then the intervention is stopped for this group and started for the other group (e.g., Devon et al. 2005). This may be suitable for interventions where it is thought the effects of the intervention on the subjects being intervened upon will decay rapidly after the intervention is stopped.

Stepped-wedge trial

In this design, the units are often in the same organization (e.g. hospital units or wards). First, one unit is exposed to the intervention; then, after a period, an additional unit is exposed so that the two units are now receiving the intervention. Then another unit is added, and so on, until all are exposed. Quite sophisticated statistical analysis is needed here (Brown and Lilford 2006). Those not receiving it act as controls, not only because they do not receive the intervention, but also because both they and the intervention units are exposed to changes other than the intervention and which may affect outcomes, such as a hospital or national campaign on safety, which might not have been predicted when the trial was started (Brown and Lilford 2006).

Observational designs

These designs are for evaluations of treatments, changes or programmes in real-world settings. The intervention/change is not planned and introduced as an experiment with careful controls, but it and the outcomes are observed. This is often done retrospectively, or concurrently with little time to plan. The designs often cost less and take less time than many experimental designs. The generalizability may be greater as the study setting is less artificial (the external validity of the study). However, certainty about outcomes being due to the intervention with these designs is often less because of fewer outcomes (the internal validity of the study).

These designs are used when controlled implementation is difficult or unethical, or when little time and few resources are available, or for other practical reasons – sometimes these designs are called 'naturalistic evaluations' where the intervention or service to be evaluated is studied 'in the wild', often as it 'evolves' in its 'environment'.

The first sub-category below is observational evaluations which collect quantitative data: usually called audit, cohort, case-control and cross-sectional designs. But these terms can be applied to describe evaluations using qualitative data as the terms describe the design, not the data collection method.

Quantitative: audit, cohort, case-control and cross-sectional evaluation designs

Audit evaluations

Some people say audits are not evaluations. It is true that some audits do not assess outcomes of a service: accreditations use audit design and, traditionally, have not considered outcomes but have assessed whether a service meets defined standards. If it does meet these standards, then it is thought that doing so contributes to achieving the desired outcomes. A clinical audit is where an assessment is made of whether practitioners or a service are meeting practice or service standards. Some audits include follow-up action as part of an 'audit cycle', but audit evaluation design is primarily about comparing what is done with what should be done – the latter usually specified as one or more standards or guidelines. The value of what is done, such as whether a hospital has a policy and procedures for identifying and reducing infections, is assessed against a specified standard of expectation, as shown in Figure 4.4.

An audit design to evaluate a primary care centre would require a description of procedures and standards for the centre programme. The evaluation would then compare these to what the centre personnel actually did, using documentation, observation and interviews. This is what many 'quality assurance' or 'compliance' evaluations do. This may be an appropriate design if users wanted to know if a service or programme was implemented according to specifications. Some implementation evaluations use this design to evaluate the 'fidelity' of the intervention to the plan or what was specified.

The assumption is that if people follow procedures, then they are doing something of value. This may be valid, for example, where it is already known that the intervention is effective and the procedures describe exactly what people should do to get the results. However, the intervention may be ineffective or the standards may not necessarily contribute to the desired outcomes. The strengths of the design are that few

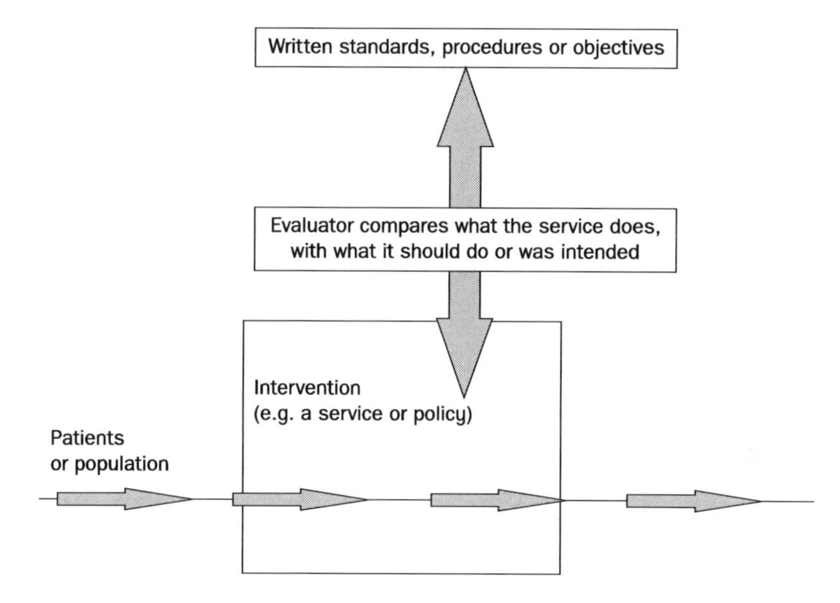

Figure 4.4 The audit cycle

resources are needed, it can be done quickly, and it is good for self-evaluation. It can help to understand why a policy or intervention fails or succeeds, and can sometimes give knowledge which can be generalized.

Cohort evaluations

Observational evaluation designs using quantitative data are usually termed 'cohort' evaluations when they collect data about the same subjects exposed to the intervention at different times.

Subjects may be chosen on the basis of high or low performance on an outcome, where the evaluation is seeking to assess what the effect of a variety of influences on the outcome may be (e.g. why are these units performing so much better than others?). The evaluator then measures different variables that might influence the outcome. Over a period of time the subjects in the sample are observed to see whether or how they develop the outcome of interest (e.g. show high performance on some indicators), and statistical analyses are used to assess which variables are associated with these outcomes.

One advantage of the cohort design is that it can be used where retrospective evaluation is required or where RCTs are unethical or impractical. It is also useful for exploring different hypotheses about the strength of different influences on outcome – if data about these variables are available. The latter points to one of the limitations of retrospective cohort evaluations – quantitative data may not be available for some possibly important influences, and informed observers' assessments are often the only data that can be gathered. Another is that if two groups are compared, it is difficult to control for all the other factors that could influence outcomes.

Cross-sectional studies and case-control studies

Cross-sectional designs are where data are collected at one time, looking across a range of subjects and are usually retrospective. This design is usually used to assess prevalence (e.g. how many personnel received the training?). Case-control evaluations are usually retrospective. People or units with the outcome of interest are matched with a control group who do not show it. Then the evaluation assesses whether they were exposed to the intervention or other influences which may explain the difference (Mann 2003; see also Dreyer et al. 2010, on observational studies for comparative effectiveness research).

Qualitative or mixed methods observational evaluation designs

The second sub-category of observational designs are those that collect qualitative data or use mixed data collection methods, sometimes called 'naturalistic approaches' to evaluation. The designs use specific techniques to maximize internal and external validity. This group of designs and these techniques are perhaps less familiar to medical and health services researchers but have a long history with social scientists, international health researchers and in health promotion/education and public health research, as well as for educational, social work, mental health and welfare programme evaluators (WHO 1981; Shadish et al. 1991; Greene 1993; JCSEE 1994; Owen and Rodgers 1999). The main sub-categories are: single case evaluation, case-comparison evaluation, and the more recent realist evaluation, each with different designs within these sub-categories.

Single case evaluation

The single case usually refers to the subject or unit receiving the intervention, which may be defined at different levels: one team, or one microsystem, or one organizational unit or system, or a region, and sometimes a nation, as in 'evaluation of X health reform'.

Take as an example an intervention to improve hand hygiene: a combination of online training, assistance to build a measurement system for feedback to providers, and financial incentives. This intervention may be directed only at a specific level (e.g. one nursing unit), and the evaluation considers its impact on the unit and other outcomes, as well as the surrounding 'context' influences which may affect implementation of the intervention (e.g. top management support, existence of IT systems which can be used for easier collection and feedback of data; Alexander et al. 2006). Or the same intervention may be directed at more than one level (e.g. a statewide intervention, run by a statewide unit) in which case the 'context' is national and local factors which may affect 'uptake' of the intervention by the lower levels in the state.

Sometimes 'the case' is the intervention, such as an intervention to patients, for example, a special stroke service with multiple components which differ from 'usual care'. The single case evaluation describes the data collection times and methods and validity techniques used to evaluate the stroke service, but without a comparison to 'usual care'. Some formative, process, outcome, or programme evaluations use this design. Part II gives examples of three types of single case observational designs (Examples 4, 6, 7). Other examples are given in Øvretveit and Aslaksen (1999); Walshe and Shortell (2004); and Øvretveit et al. (2012).

Keen and Packwood (1995) describe case study evaluation (CSE) as:

> valuable where broad, complex questions have to be addressed in complex circumstances . . . when the question being posed requires an investigation of a real life intervention in detail, where the focus is on how and why the intervention succeeds or fails, where the general context will influence the outcome and where researchers asking the questions will have no control over events. As a result, the number of relevant variables will be far greater than can be controlled for, so that experimental approaches are simply not appropriate.

CSE is useful where an intervention is not well defined or standardizable and cannot easily be distinguished from the general environment, or where it involves a number of components, each of which may change over time. Rather than assessing efficacy, CSEs are more useful for describing and explaining implementation, a variety of intermediate outcomes, and for addressing questions concerning adoption, spread and sustainability. For evidence and for explanations of intermediate and patient outcomes, many CSEs use triangulation of data – combining data from different sources to see if the same pattern is reflected in different data. The data often include informants' estimations about whether and what effects the intervention had.

The degree of certainty about whether the intervention results in intermediate or final outcomes is less than for experimental designs because confounders and competing explanations are not controlled for and cannot be excluded. However, if other influences apart from the intervention are recognized and their influence understood (e.g. environmental factors), a case study design can help build an understanding of how both the intervention and the environment contribute to intermediate and final outcomes, as well as knowledge about implementation.

Case evaluation designs vary in the type of pre-data collection work which different designs undertake. Some use minimal pre-planning of which data to collect, and focus on documenting and describing the changes planned and made as the intervention is implemented, before then deciding which data to collect to discover different types of intermediate and later outcomes, or to check if intended outcomes have been achieved. More often, and increasingly, case evaluations use theory to define which data to collect about which outcomes (Bickman 2008). This can be a theory of how actions in the programme will lead to certain results, which allows the evaluators to identify which data to collect to assess if the actions are carried out, and which indicators or data may show intended or theorized outcomes at different stages (the programme theory or logic model of the intervention; Shekelle et al. 2010).

Case comparison evaluation

This is like the above-noted 'cohort' design, but uses the validity-enhancing strategies for qualitative data and mixed methods of the single case evaluation just mentioned, such as triangulation and programme theory. Part II presents Example 5, which is an evaluation of a large-scale safety programme that compared each of four hospitals receiving the programme with other hospitals not receiving the programme (Benning et al. 2011). Another example is a comparison of two case hospitals, each of which received an intervention to implement an electronic medical record (Øvretveit et al. 2007). This case comparison evaluation used previous research into similar interventions to pre-define which data to collect to test hypotheses from earlier studies about which aspects of the intervention were necessary for effective implementation.

Realist evaluation

These designs identify context-mechanism-outcome (CMO) configurations in complex interventions in different settings, and aim to establish 'what works for whom in which settings' (Pawson and Tilley 1997). The assumption, based on some evidence from education and criminal programmes, is that, in social interventions, outcomes are a function of both 'the mechanism' through which the intervention works and the context in which it is applied: there are different effects in different settings, even if the same intervention is used. Part II gives one example of an evaluation of a large-scale 'transformation' of health services in London which uses this design, and describes its strengths and weaknesses in Chapter 8.

The aim is not only to describe the intervention but to clarify the 'generative mechanism': this is the essential idea or 'active ingredient' which is the basis for the intervention (e.g. performance feedback). Using this approach, superficially different interventions can be grouped and compared through their underlying logic. Another aim is to examine how much and how the mechanism depends on, or interacts with, the context to produce different effects.

The design uses a programme model or theory (sometimes called a logic model) to select programmes and test hypotheses about the CMO configuration for one intervention in one setting. Then the design studies programmes theorized as 'similar' in other settings to examine how the interactions between C, M and O vary. Interventions are viewed as 'theories in practice'. Discovering poor or no outcomes for a similar intervention in a different setting is an opportunity to refine the logic model of the CMO configuration.

This approach thus emphasizes studying, in a variety of situations, the mechanism which is thought to generate certain results: this might be embodied in interventions which appear to be quite different. The approach is similar to a case study evaluation in describing and understanding outcomes as the product of an intervention implementation in an environment. However, it differs from some case study evaluations in emphasizing the logic model testing and the comparison between different implementations, as well as in elucidating the essential features of the mechanism to allow a comparison of a variety of superficially different changes.

One possible limitation is that the concepts of context, mechanism and outcome are not easy to define and are only illustrated in a few studies. It is also unclear exactly how 'mechanism' is elucidated in such studies: 'mechanism' does not just refer to the intervention components or implementing actions, but also how this higher-level conceptualization of 'mechanism' is created is unclear, in terms of how the actions 'work' ('the generative mechanism'), which is different from their interaction with the context. Examples of studies using these methods to study safety, quality or other interventions to organizations include: Redfern et al. (2002); Blaise and Kegels (2004); Byng et al. (2005, 2008). Some limitations are described in Davis (2005).

Evaluating innovations in healthcare delivery and digital health technologies (DHT)

> The complexity of innovation makes it unsuitable for experimental evaluation design (Booth and Falzon 2001; Berwick 2008). In order to capture the range of individual, group and organizational level processes and outcomes, a combination of approaches might be adopted. For example, qualitative individual reflections, evaluation of group process through action research and quality assurance in relation to organizational processes.
>
> (Williams 2011)

Action evaluation designs

> If you show implementers data from your evaluation while they are implementing the intervention, they might change what they would otherwise do. And others later using this intervention may not have researchers to give them feedback while they are implementing it, so they may get different results.

Both these points are true, but if the user wants feedback from an evaluation to help develop or implement the intervention, then designs within this category meet their needs. And for some interventions, collecting data about results and giving reviews of and adjustments to the intervention are part of the intervention and integral to its implementation – they are iterative corrections to make it effective in a particular environment. A simple example is trying new text or colour on a website and then looking at whether readers stay longer or shorter there than before. In this sense, evaluation is not separate from implementation and development.

Are these designs different from the other two categories of design? No – at least in many senses, they are not different: all of the designs described above can be used in an action evaluation. That is, apart from the obvious difference: the evaluator gives their data or feedback to the implementers at some time, or continuously as part of the implementation. Through this, they may change the content of the intervention or the implementation in some way, which they need to document. This would be shown on any of the above design diagrams as one or more arrows at certain times showing the evaluator giving feedback.

One assumption is that if the evaluation is useful to different parties during rather than after the evaluation, then evaluators can gain information and insights which they may not otherwise gain. By collaborating and participating in the shaping of the intervention, they may be better able to document how it has changed and why, and be better able to explain later findings.

The limitations of action evaluation, compared to experimental designs, are to both the internal and external validity of the evaluation. In fact, this is more so than the qualitative case evaluations described above, because of the participatory role of the researcher. These limitations are the compromise in this approach by the greater explanatory power gained by researchers from their action researcher role and participation.

One challenge is to assess the role and impact of the researchers, in order that others are able to judge whether they need a similar input if they were to implement a similar intervention, either from other researchers or internal or external experts. Sometimes action evaluation is suitable for the development phases of the intervention, or for an intervention which is likely to require significant modification in order to be implemented.

Varieties of action evaluation

In some respects, formative evaluations are action evaluations because the evaluator provides an analysis to the implementers or intervention designers which helps them 'form' the intervention. Greenhalgh et al.'s (2009) realist evaluation described in Part II is an action evaluation, and formative to the transformation programme evaluated. A distinguishing feature of different designs within this category is whether feedback occurs once only or a few times, or continuously, and how integrated the evaluation is with the implementation.

One variant of an action evaluation is being used in the variety of action evaluation to develop and evaluate the variety of action evaluation version of the patient-centred medical home. Related to an earlier approach, termed 'evidence-based quality improvement' (EBQI) (Rubenstein et al. 2006, 2010), this approach involves the researchers assisting primary healthcare personnel in a number of ways to design and implement changes (providing evidence of effective practice, training in quality improvement methods) and to report findings from the evaluation to the implementers.

This 'EBQI' approach is one of a new range of action evaluations emerging to meet a demand from research funders and providers for more timely and relevant research. These new evaluation methods blur the boundaries between implementers and evaluators. Evaluators increasingly use data already collected by the growing number of electronic databases to carry out real-time research in learning health systems (IOM

2007; Friedman et al. 2010; Pearson et al. 2011; Academy Health 2012; Riley et al. 2013). For more details, the best simple overview of action evaluation is a section in Robson (1993), and for a more comprehensive overview, see Waterman et al. (2001) (see also Hart and Bond 1996 and Øvretveit 2002).

Conclusion

Design shows which data are collected and the main features of the evaluation in order to plan it and communicate it. This chapter has described a range of designs to help choose one which is most suited to the evaluation users' information needs and to the time, money, skills and data that are already available.

Experimental designs focus on whether the intervention causes changes in a few measurable outcomes of interest, and use different methods to exclude 'confounders'. Observation or naturalistic approaches examine more variables or influences but are not able to establish the same type of certainty about associations, and sometimes conceive of the intervention as part of a system of influences. Some naturalistic approaches do not standardize the intervention but describe how it is implemented and how different local and broader factors affect implementation. They also document a variety of intermediate outcomes and impacts. As such, they are suited to questions about impact and implementation (including adoption, spread and sustainability). Action evaluations aim to provide early feedback from the evaluation to enable implementers to improve the intervention and its implementation. There is rapid innovation in action evaluation methods due to the variety of clinical and other data available and analysable, using new software, and to some recognizing the value of 'good-enough' evaluation for rapid improvements and real-time evaluations.

More details of different designs and their strengths and weaknesses can be found in Robson (1993); Øvretveit (1998, 2002); Tunis et al. (2003); Craig et al. (2007); Mercer et al. (2007); and Fan et al. (2010).

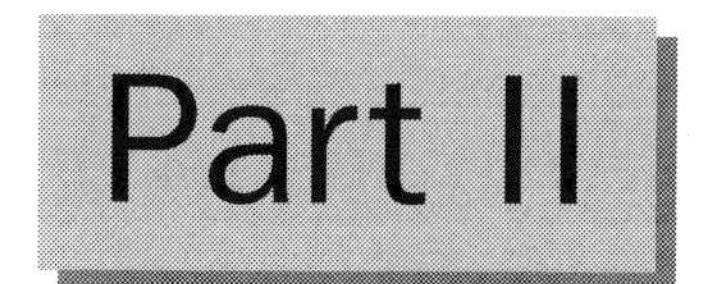

Part II Introduction: Example evaluations – do they answer users' questions?

Example evaluations and practical advice

Part II looks at whether the design chosen by an example evaluation was able to meet users' needs. It discusses the strengths and weaknesses of different designs for these purposes, and gives further advice on how to plan and carry out an evaluation.

The chapters are divided into discussions of evaluations, first, of interventions to patients (Chapter 5), then interventions to professionals (Chapter 6), and then interventions to services and service performance (Chapter 7). The final two chapters look at evaluations of interventions to health systems and then of interventions to populations (Chapters 8 and 9).

Why consider examples of evaluations in this way, in terms of the subjects of the interventions? These entities or subjects which are intended to benefit from the intervention are obviously different: patients, professionals, health services, health systems and populations. All the evaluation approaches and designs described in Chapter 4 can, in principle, be used to evaluate interventions to each of these types of subject. But the nature of the change which most interventions seek to engender in each of these subjects is different. Enabling a person to change, for example, by giving medication or helping them change their diet and lifestyle is not the same as enabling a professional to change their behaviour or increase their knowledge. There is some overlap, but the professional culture and work setting are different for professionals than the environment which affects patient interventions.

Health services are social organizations that are unique in their nature and different to human individuals. The methods to evaluate interventions to social organizations are also different from those for evaluating interventions to individuals. These differences and their significance are explained in the introduction to each chapter.

The data collected to describe a standard intervention to a patient will not be the same as those data collected to describe an intervention to a health system or to a population. Also, as we move from patients to higher-complexity social organizations, such as health systems and populations, we see that some designs become less feasible for evaluating interventions to these entities, such as the randomized controlled trial (RCT) design. Which design to choose depends on the users' questions, and there are different questions to be answered by evaluations of interventions to these different entities.

Each chapter also considers evaluation designs for performance evaluation. This is where no intervention as such is being evaluated, but the performance of individuals or programmes is being assessed, usually by comparing them to others. Examples are performance evaluations of individual practitioners, or of healthcare services through accreditation designs or performance indicator system designs.

The chapters in Part II also show the use of the ADAGU method to assess the strengths and weaknesses of evaluations considered, in relation to these five questions:

- *Aims*: what information is needed and what are the questions to be addressed?
- *Description*: what are the details of the intervention, its implementation and the context?
- *Attribution*: how confident can we be that the intervention caused the outcomes reported?
- *Generalization*: can we copy it and obtain similar results?
- *Usefulness*: in which situations are the intervention and implementation feasible and how do we enable users to use the findings from the evaluation?

The designs used are those described in Chapter 4. Here we summarize the key points of an evaluation presented in the chapters in Part II:

1 The purpose of the evaluation and its question
2 The intervention evaluated
3 The design
4 Outcomes measured and discovered
5 Certainty about the outcomes
6 Generalizability (of the intervention, and of the evaluation findings, if the intervention were to be implemented elsewhere in the same way)
7 Strengths and weaknesses for answering the question.

Designs considered

Examples of the different designs used in real evaluations are given in the chapters in Part II and the list below details where each type of evaluation example is given.

Randomized controlled trial design

- Chapter 5, Example 3: RCT of the care transitions intervention
- Chapter 7, Example 7: Pragmatic cluster RCT of a multifaceted intervention to 15 intensive care units

Quasi-experimental design

- Chapter 5, Example 2: Before/after evaluation of Guatemalan doll therapy
- Chapter 6, Example 5: Interrupted time series evaluation of a hand hygiene intervention
- Chapter 9: Comparative trial: Example evaluation of an intervention to a community to prevent heart disease

Observational design

- Chapter 6, Example 4: Mixed methods prospective observational evaluation of an intervention to change primary care physicians' behaviour
- Chapter 6, Example 6: Process evaluation of an intervention to promote smoking cessation
- Chapter 7, Example 8: Mixed methods, prospective, observational evaluation of large-scale safety programme
- Chapter 7, Example 9: Case evaluation of a programme for electronic summaries of patients' medical records (mixed methods)

Action evaluation

- Chapter 8, Example 10: Formative realist case evaluation design: of large-scale transformation of health services in London

Evaluating performance

- Chapter 5, Example 3: Patients' performance, for example, in self-care performance
- Chapter 6: Practitioner performance, for example, in communicating with patients
- Chapter 7: Service performance, for example, in relation to quality standards
- Chapter 8: Health system performance, for example, in meeting the triple aim for population health (Stiefel and Nolan 2012)
- Chapter 9: Public health service or health promotion programme performance

Other examples and designs not considered here are discussed in Øvretveit (1998 and 2002).

5 Evaluating interventions to patients and patient performance

Introduction

We have all helped someone when they were ill. We intervened to change what otherwise would have happened. But what difference did our help make? There were many outcomes, in addition to those we intended. An evaluation can only concentrate on a few outcomes, and on finding out if these did, in fact, 'come out' of our help.

The aims of this chapter are to show how different designs for evaluating interventions to patients answer different questions, as well as illustrating designs in three example evaluations. It also aims to give simple and quick ways to understand an evaluation and judge its validity for your purposes. This is done by asking and answering the few questions in the discussion section after each evaluation is presented.

How to evaluate patient performance?

In addition to showing how to evaluate interventions, other chapters show how to evaluate performance such as physician performance or service performance. But in which sense would anyone want to evaluate the performance of a patient? And why do so?

There is increasing awareness that what patients do to take care of themselves is, for many illnesses or for after-surgery periods, crucial to their health and to prevent deterioration. Methods for assessing a patient's performance in their own self-care are forms of evaluation. There is no intervention which these methods evaluate, though these methods are used in evaluations of interventions to improve self-care capacity, such as in the evaluations of educational programmes delivered on the internet.

Mostly, this chapter gives examples of healthcare evaluations of interventions made to patients. These evaluations have generally been carried out on a variety of topics, such as drugs, other treatments, and diagnostic methods. Also, there have been evaluations of practitioners' help to patients, and of entire 'service packages' which arrange a number of types of intervention to patients, and sometimes to their family or friends' informal care system.

The chapter starts with an example of a simple evaluation using a before/after design (Example 1). It notes some of the challenges and solutions in evaluating interventions to patients. Then it presents Example 2 and demonstrates a simple five-question method for quickly understanding an evaluation, and shows the comparative trial design used in the evaluation. Example 3 is an evaluation of a complex intervention to improve the transition of patients from hospital to home, using a randomized controlled trial design. Then we consider why and how to evaluate patient performance.

Example 1 Does Guatemalan doll therapy work?

Kerstin excitedly showed me a small doll, 2 cm from top to toe. She began to get serious when I laughed and patiently explained to me that this was a special doll from Guatemala. But more – if you told your doll your worries, then your worries would go away.

Kerstin's mother explained that, when she or her daughters had trouble sleeping, they put the doll under their pillow and they found that they could sleep better. 'We know the value of our Guatemalan dolls, and they work for us, but I bet your scientific evaluation methods would say that they do not. How would you evaluate our dolls, then?'

I will not tell you how the discussion went, but I will ask you to test what you know about evaluation on this example. We will look at one of the simplest quasi-experimental designs: the before/after design. We have an intervention, which we can call 'Guatemalan doll therapy' (GDT). We could evaluate its effects on reducing worries – after all, that was what Kerstin claimed. Let us keep it simple and evaluate it as a way of helping with sleeplessness, because this is easier to measure.

Interest group perspectives

'How would you evaluate it, then?' was the challenge. In the situation above, I instinctively reached for the academic's answer when needing time to think: 'It depends.' A moment's thought and I realized that this was the right answer, because the starting point for any evaluation is to clarify for whom we are evaluating the item. As described earlier, the purpose of evaluation is to help people to make better-informed decisions – we need to understand what they need to know for them to act differently. People have different questions which relate to the decisions they have to make in their social roles.

We could evaluate an intervention like GDT from six different perspectives, each with a different set of questions, and different actions by each group would follow from an informed answer to the questions. Normally we would design our evaluation to answer the questions of one or more interest groups or 'users' of the evaluation, and we would use a different design for different questions.

Patients' values

In the example, we will not take the perspective of Kerstin's mother and sisters: they believe GDT works, and their theory that it reduces sleeplessness is built on their experience. But other people who do not sleep well have questions which they would like answered before they are prepared to go to the trouble of getting a doll and trying it for themselves. We can call people who go to a health service for help with their sleeping problem 'patients'. Patients' questions are 'Does it work?', and, if it does, 'How well does it work?' They may already use other therapies and, if GDT 'works', they may want to know how well it works in comparison to sleeping pills or other common sleeplessness strategies, like counting sheep or salmon jumping up a stream.

If we were doing an evaluation only for this interest group or from its perspective, we would then pursue things further with these 'evaluation users'. We would try to focus on the most important questions by looking at whether answers to each question would lead people to act differently or not. This would help us to separate the 'interesting questions' from those of real consequence for their lives, and to focus on the latter. We would also define the criteria which they use to judge the value of the therapy, for example, reducing sleeplessness, effort involved and no side effects. We would use these criteria of valuation to decide which outcome variables to measure and data to collect.

If we were to use an experimental perspective, we would also translate patients' questions into 'theories' or hypotheses to test, for example, 'Using GDT has no effect whatsoever on sleeplessness.' But all of this is jumping ahead to later parts of the chapter. It may be that other patients would feel that their answers would be satisfied by a detailed description of how Kerstin, her sisters and mother use GDT and of their experience. At present, however, we need to decide whether the patient's perspective is the only one we will take in designing the evaluation. Who else would have an interest in an evaluation of GDT for sleeplessness? Who else might be 'users' of the evaluation and what questions would they want the evaluation to answer?

Practitioners' values

A second set of potential users are healthcare workers whom people suffering from sleeplessness consult for help, such as nurses or doctors. If you were a doctor or nurse who had heard about this therapy, what questions would you have of an evaluation of GDT? What would you need to know which would make you act differently? Because doctors and nurses understand their patients' concerns, we would expect them to have similar questions to patients, but they would want stronger evidence than a detailed report of one family's experience: 'Does it work for all patients with this problem?' They will also have questions about side effects, about long-term effects and about interactions with other therapies which some of their patients might be undergoing.

Managers' values

A third interest group is managers, such as the managers of primary healthcare centres or of a health financing agency. What questions would they have of an evaluation of GDT? 'How much does it cost?' and 'How much could it save us?' are probably their main questions. They would also want answers to questions like those raised by the doctors, if only to give a credible explanation to healthcare workers about why they were, or were not, supporting the introduction of GDT therapy in their service – they expect patients' groups to demand it and expect healthcare workers to criticize them for trying to save money. They are also interested in possible risks, because their service might be blamed for giving a treatment which could cause harm.

Payers' values

A fourth interest group perspective which we could take account of in the evaluation is that of payers. These are often people other than the patient – insurers or tax-payers represented by politicians. Politicians have to make choices about how much money to allocate to different purposes, and must justify these choices. Their social role also requires them to be sensitive to and respond to the wishes of the people they represent. They also want to be re-elected and want to look good to the section of the population on whose vote they depend. They have similar questions to patients, doctors and managers, but with a different emphasis and priority: they are concerned about cost-effectiveness because they will have to defend their decisions, but they also want to know, 'How many people want it and which people?' If they are also responsible for social and educational services, they will want to know if there are any extra costs or benefits for these services and possible wider effects.

Academics' values

A fifth interest group are scientists and health researchers. Their questions are, 'What is already known about this or similar therapies?', 'What are the effects?' and 'Why do any effects occur? What are the causes of any effects?' An evaluation for this group would require a different, and probably more costly, design from that which would answer the questions of other groups.

The media

Last but not least is the sixth group which evaluators have to bear in mind: journalists and 'the media'. In theory, they represent the general public who have questions about the best use of their money as tax-payers. In practice, they are looking for a good story and for drama. This group is not an interest group with a perspective in the same way that the other groups are in that there is less commonality of interest. However, evaluators need to consider their questions and how the media might use the evaluation, especially if one or more of the media are sponsoring the evaluation.

Implementation of the results of an evaluation is more likely if the evaluation has paid attention to the concerns and questions of interest groups which can support or oppose changes. These are the six groups which are often significant in any action following an evaluation study. There will be different sub-interests and perspectives within each group.

There are other interest group perspectives which the evaluation might take into account, such as those of drug companies, social welfare departments and employers. However, the main point highlighted here is that the perspective which the evaluation takes decides which questions it will aim to answer and the type of design which is best for answering them, given the time and resources available.

'How would you evaluate it, then?' When faced with this question from Kerstin's mother, I was able to explain that it depended on for whom I was doing the evaluation. I then wanted to start talking about how we could tell if it worked or not and to use some evaluation concepts, but I could see things were getting too abstract. I decided to do what many people do when asked how they would evaluate this treatment – go straight to talking about evaluation designs and leave the explanation of technical terms until later.

What is in the box?

Using the paper and cultured pen which Kerstin put on the kitchen table, I drew the 'basic diagram' shown in Figure 5.1. I explained to Kerstin that the box is the 'doll therapy'. The arrow shows people who do not use the doll before, and then they use it and are inside the box, and then they stop using it, and move outside of the box. 'But I use it all the time', protested Kerstin. 'OK, then we will not close the box – we will take the line out and instead of after, we will put "later" to show data are collected after using the doll for a bit.' 'What?' said Kerstin. 'How long after?' said her sister. Things were not going well. I thought the picture would have explained it.

'Why do people go inside the box?' asked Kerstin. 'They just do', I said, but this did not satisfy Kerstin's mother. 'Well, it is to show that people "go through" the intervention. In the evaluation business we say that they are the "targets" who are "exposed" to the intervention.' Kerstin looked troubled. 'Why do people stop using the doll when it works?' 'So that we can find out if it works.' 'Why . . .' 'They just do', I interrupted, asking Kerstin for another piece of paper so that I could draw different designs.

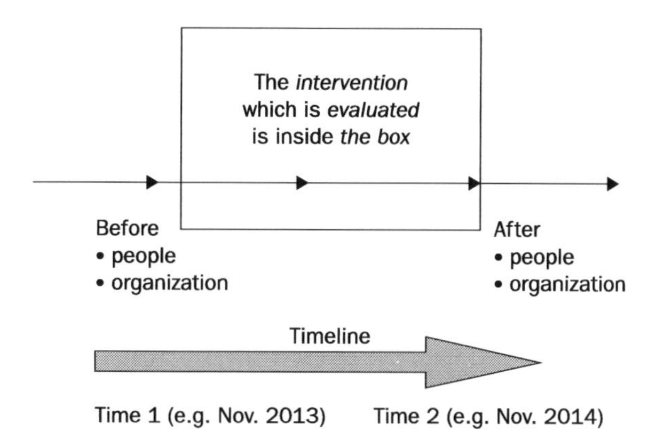

Figure 5.1 The box design diagram of the GDT intervention

I need to say at this point that, unknown to Kerstin and her family, an evaluation had already been done – it is summarized below.

A summary of the evaluation of GDT

According to Astra and Littlejohn (1993, pp. 13–14):

> Extravagant claims have been made for Guatemalan Doll Therapy as a cure for sleeplessness and other ailments, but there is little reported evidence of effectiveness. Concern was raised by Astra and Littlejohn (1993) that the use of this treatment might delay diagnosis of underlying depression, which could be further exacerbated if the treatment failed. In the evaluation reported in this paper, 20 patients from a primary health care centre in Bergen, Norway, were selected for treatment using this method. The patients were all members of the Norwegian West Coast Sleeplessness Society, which sponsored the evaluation.

The treatment consisted of patients telling their worries to a 2-cm high Guatemalan doll purchased from a distributor in Gothenburg, Sweden. The patients were instructed to tell their worries to the doll for no less than five minutes just before bed, and afterwards to place the doll under their pillow as described in the instructions given with the doll. They were instructed to do this every night for four weeks. The length of uninterrupted sleep was measured over a five-day period before the treatment, and then during the fourth week of treatment for a five-day period. The method of measurement and recording was the patient noting the time of uninterrupted sleep in a diary in the morning.

The findings were that seven patients slept longer on average during the five days in the fourth week of treatment than they did for the five days before treatment. All seven slept longer than six hours uninterrupted on each night. Over the five days before treatment three reported less than four hours' uninterrupted sleep for two nights and four reported less than five hours' uninterrupted sleep for three nights. No significant difference in uninterrupted sleep was reported by the ten other patients for whom measures were available.

The study shows that some benefit was reported by seven out of 17 patients and that Guatemalan doll therapy might be a cost-effective treatment for some types of sleep disorder.

Discussion of the evaluation example

What were the strengths and weaknesses of this evaluation of an intervention to patients? Many are the strengths and weaknesses of the before/after design. But some are due to the way this design was applied, such as which data were collected and how other explanations for outcomes were considered. There is a simple five-question assessment method that can be used to make sense of any evaluation. Here we use these simple five questions to help understand the GDT:

1 *What was evaluated?*

Telling worries to a 'Guatemalan doll' for at least five minutes before bed, and putting the doll under your pillow.

2 *What were the comparisons?*

This is the length of sleep of ten people before and after three weeks of starting the treatment.

3 *What were the measures or the data which were gathered?*

This is the length of uninterrupted sleep as noted by patients in their diaries in the morning.

4 *What were the criteria of valuation?*

This is not stated explicitly, but, given the measures used, the criteria for valuation appear to be uninterrupted sleep, harmful effects and cost, although data were only gathered about the first.

5 *Which design did the evaluation use?*

It used the 'before and after' comparison of change in one measure (Figure 5.2).

Strengths and limitations of the evaluation

Some of the things to consider when assessing how well the design and the evaluation serve their purpose, and how useful they are to your decisions, are:

1 Is it clear or implied who are to be the users of the evaluation?
2 Is it clear which decisions and actions the evaluation is intended to inform?

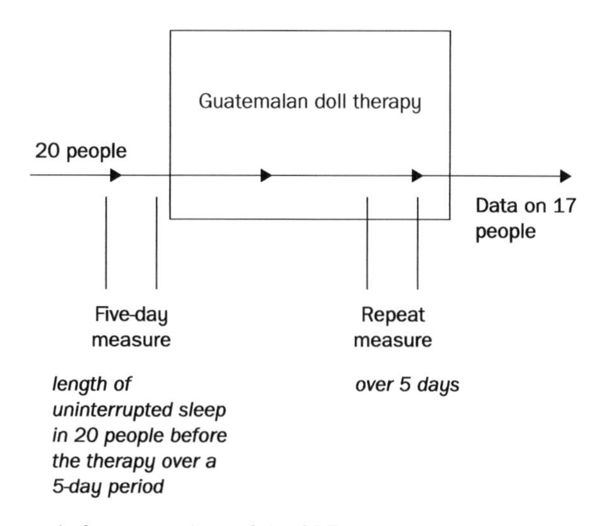

Figure 5.2 Before and after comparison of the GDT

3 Was there bias in the sample, in selection before, and in the population measured after (i.e. drop-outs)?
4 Would the study have detected possibly important unintended effects?
5 What changes might the evaluation itself have produced which reduce the validity of the findings?
6 What are the strengths and weaknesses of the data-gathering methods/measures for the purpose?
7 Were all the limitations described?
8 Were the conclusions justified by the results?
9 Could some people be misled by the report?
10 Would the conclusions be credible to the audience for the evaluation (the users)?
11 Were there any unethical aspects?
12 Could the purpose have been achieved with fewer resources or in a shorter time?

Below is one assessment made by answering these questions.

Strengths

As a simple and low-cost evaluation for a patients' association, the evaluation does have some strengths, but the purpose of the evaluation is implied rather than stated. The strengths are that objective measures were attempted of one type of outcome (uninterrupted sleep), which have some validity and the findings could support a proposal for a more rigorous evaluation.

Limitations

It is not stated clearly who the evaluation is for or its purpose. No clear questions or hypotheses were set. The decisions or actions which the evaluation could inform are implied rather than stated in the conclusion. The treatment is not well-defined and other causes of interruptions to sleep are not controlled. It would have been possible to define a hypothesis for this type of study, which would have strengthened and focused it: for example, 'use of GDT has no effect on length of uninterrupted sleep over a five-day period, four weeks after the treatment is started.'

Bias may have been introduced in the selection of patients and in the group for whom data were available, but no details were given. The sample size was small. No attempt was made to discover harmful effects, or whether any effects were sustained with or without the treatment. The summary did not describe the limitations of the design or of the data collection methods. It is not clear what the evaluators consider a 'significant difference' in uninterrupted sleep in ten patients. The size of the difference in uninterrupted sleep for the seven patients who benefited was not clearly presented.

Other comments

The evaluation is of some use even though it has many weaknesses. It is difficult to see how it could have been done better with the same time and resources without knowing the purpose, which has to be inferred. It also raises interesting questions about how to design an evaluation which would be more conclusive and have more credibility with health professionals, if more finance were available. Should the possible effect of the treatment on other types of sleep problem be investigated? Should patients be interviewed to discover their views of the treatment? How would such a design control for other possible causes or explanations of interruptions to sleep? Can and should a placebo be used to control for some factors? Some of these questions can best be answered by clarifying the purpose of a future evaluation, but there are some questions which might not be answerable by using an experimental evaluation technique for evaluating this type of treatment.

Which of my comments do you disagree with? Note: there is one 'deliberate mistake' (a comment which is not correct).

Example 2 What is the health value of prescribing exercise?

This example is of an evaluation of an intervention to patients of a different type: a prescription for exercise. After the summary, a reminder and demonstration of the simple five-question method for quickly understanding an evaluation are presented.

> A national fitness survey in the UK in 1991 showed the health problems of inactivity, and a number of studies have reported the health benefits of increased exercise. However, health practitioners have not found it easy to get people to take more exercise. In this study GPs referred patients to one of two local health centres for a 'prescription' of a ten-week gym exercise programme (Lockwood 1994). Patients paid £1.50 per session at the Selby centre and £1 at York, and could also use other facilities, such as the swimming pool. Patients were offered reduced rates for joining the gym after the programme to encourage their continued attendance at the centre: 50 per cent did so at Selby and 67 per cent at York. The only health service financing was £300, which was used to pay for a heart monitor for each of the two centres.

Thirty-six patients took part in the Selby scheme and 108 in the York scheme. The evaluation made a number of physical measures of each patient before and after the ten-week programme, and asked each patient to fill in a questionnaire at the start, at the end and at three and six months after the end of the exercise programme. The findings show a significant reduction in percentage body fat, body mass index and systolic blood pressure, and increases in peak flow. Overall, 91 per cent reported benefiting from the scheme and many reported improvements in self-confidence, feelings of well-being and lower levels of stress. Nine per cent reported that they did not benefit.

The number of patients completing their prescription and joining the gym (67 per cent at York) suggests that GPs are powerful motivators for change, and that this scheme is a good way to covert previously sedentary individuals into regular exercisers. A country-wide evaluation of similar schemes was published by Jackson (1997).

Five questions quickly to understand an evaluation

1 What was evaluated?
2 What were the comparisons?
3 What were the measures or the data which were gathered?
4 What were the criteria of valuation?
5 Which of the six designs did the evaluation use?

Understanding the prescribing exercise evaluation

We can apply the five-question method to understand Example 2 evaluation:

1 *What was evaluated?*

An exercise programme at community sports centres, where GPs referred patients and gave a general prescription for exercise. The summary does not give the details of the exercise programme. In fact, two separate schemes were evaluated, one at York and one at Selby.

2 *What were the comparisons?*

Before and after measures of physical characteristics of people who were referred, as well as patients' views. The two schemes were not compared – at least not in the summary report.

3 *What were the measures or the data which were gathered?*

Continued attendance at the centre after the programme, measures of body fat, body mass index, systolic blood pressure and peak flow rates before and after. Patients' answers to questions were also gathered before and at intervals after, but these data were not described in detail, apart from '91 per cent reported benefiting from the scheme, and 9 per cent reported that they did not benefit, with many reporting improvements in self-confidence, feelings of well-being and lower levels of stress.' The summary did not say at what time after the programme these reports were made.

4 *What were the criteria of valuation?*

Not stated explicitly, but the criteria for valuation appear to be whether people continued attendance, as well as changes to physical characteristics thought to reduce risks of ill health, 'patient' satisfaction and cost.

5 *Which of the six designs did the evaluation use?*

The prescribing exercise in Example 2 used a comparative experimental design (Figure 5.3).

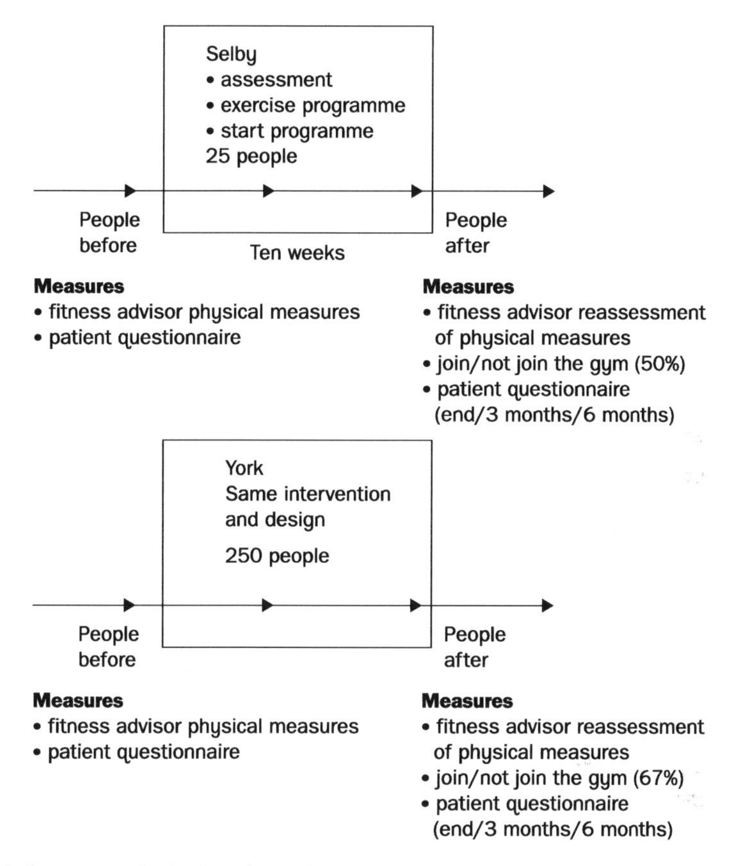

Figure 5.3 Case example design of exercise intervention

Example 3 Evaluation of a 'care transitions intervention'

Does a randomized controlled trial (RCT) design solve the problems of the before/after designs? We will see that it has fewer limitations as regards certainty of attribution, but has its own weaknesses, all depending on the purpose of the evaluation. In this example we will consider the RCT design applied to evaluate a complex 'service package' called the 'care transitions intervention' (from Coleman et al. 2006) in the USA. Most care transitions interventions have as their subject health professionals: this one aims to enable both professionals and patients better to manage transitions in care.

Summary of an RCT of a care transitions intervention

The question addressed was: 'What is the effect on re-hospitalization and hospital costs of an intervention which coaches chronically-ill older patients and their caregivers and includes a "transitions coach"?' The intervention evaluated was a combination of these elements:

- tools to promote cross-site communication including a personal health record;
- encouragement to take a more active role in their care and to assert their preferences;
- continuity across settings and guidance from a 'transition coach' (Table 5.1).

Key features of the design were that 750 older patients were admitted to the study hospital and randomly allocated to the intervention and a control group (Figure 5.4).

Table 5.1 Care transitions intervention activities by pillar and stage of intervention

	Four Pillars			
Stage of Intervention	**Medication Self-management**	**Patient-Centered Record**	**Follow-up**	**Red Flags**
Goal	Patient is knowledgeable about medications and has medication management system	Patient understands and uses PHR to facilitate communication and to ensure continuity of care plan across providers and settings; patient manages PHR	Patient schedules and completes follow-up visit with primary care provider or specialist and is prepared to be an active participant in interactions	Patient is knowledgeable about indications that condition is worsening and how to respond
Hospital visit	Discuss importance of knowing medications and having a system in place to ensure adherence to regimen	Explain PHR	Recommend primary care provider follow-up visit	Discuss symptoms and drug reactions
Home visit	Reconcile prehospitalization and posthospitalization medication lists Identify and correct discrepancies	Review and update PHR Review discharge summary Encourage patient to update and share PHR with primary care provider or specialist at follow-up visits	Emphasize importance of follow-up visit and need to provide primary care provider with recent hospitalization information Practice and role-play questions for primary care provider	Assess condition Discuss symptoms and adverse effects of medications
Follow-up telephone calls	Answer remaining medication questions	Remind patient to share PHR with primary care provider or specialist Discuss outcome of visit with primary care provider or specialist	Provide advocacy in getting appointment, if necessary	Reinforce when primary care provider should be telephoned

Source: Coleman et al. (2006).

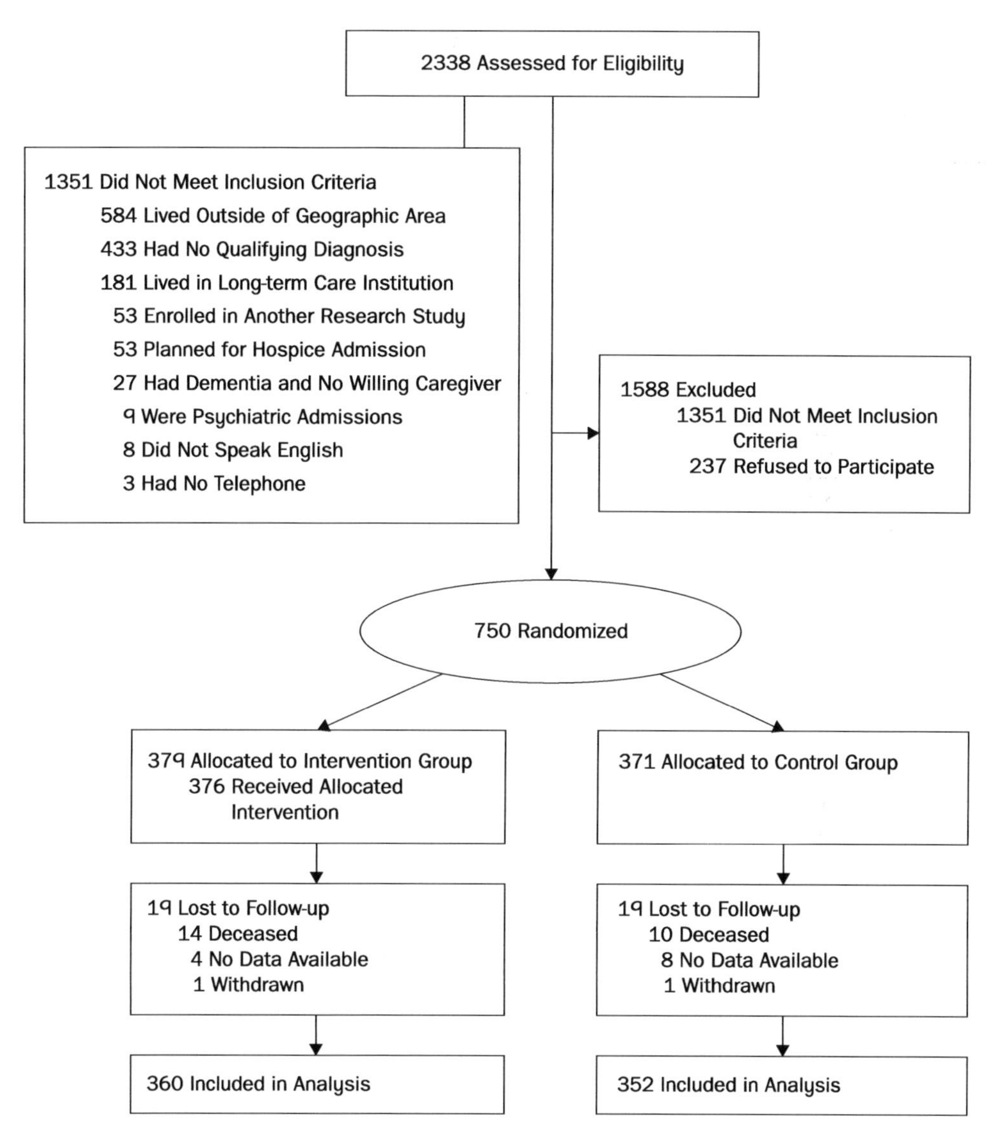

Figure 5.4 Allocation to the RCT

Source: Coleman et al. (2006).

The measures were:

- Re-hospitalization at 30, 90, 180 days (data abstracted from the study delivery system's administrative records).
- Non-elective hospital cost outcomes at 30, 90, 180 days.

The findings were that the intervention group showed lower re-hospitalization rates and lower mean hospital costs ($2058) vs. controls ($2546) at 180 days. As regards certainty about and generalizability of the outcomes, an analysis showed no significant differences between the key characteristics of the intervention group (n = 379) and the control group (n = 371), so it is unlikely that the better results for the intervention group were due to any characteristics of the patients rather than their response to the intervention, all other things being equal.

Other explanations for the findings could have been a systematic chance difference between the two groups in the primary care and after-care services they received: to some extent, this was minimized as all were covered by the same delivery system.

As regards generalization (reproducibility of the intervention and then the outcomes), the intervention could, in principle, be reproduced with more details about the different components. The results, though, might be different as in other places the primary care and after-care may be different in a way that affects the impact on the intervention.

Strengths and limitations of the design in this example

The strengths of the RCT are illustrated in this evaluation as being able to give a high certainty about the outcome findings because the patient characteristics and some other influences on outcome were controlled for. The design forces a focus on a few measures, and in this case it chooses measures and data-gathering methods for these measures which could answer the research question: the data were reasonably accessible at low cost and were valid measures for the question.

The limitations are the resources and effort to enforce the trial protocol of carefully selected patients, and to ensure the fidelity of implementation to a prescribed intervention. The measurement was costly and difficult to reproduce in other settings. The implementation steps and the details of the intervention can be described in the trial report to give others guidance to reproduce the intervention, but reproducing it is still not always easy. These are the reasons why, though the RCT gives high 'internal validity' (the certainty referred to above), the 'external validity' (generalizability) is low, unless trials are done in many settings, which is usually too expensive and time-consuming.

Evaluating patients' performance

We close this chapter by considering some of the growing number of methods for evaluating a patient's performance. What would it mean to evaluate the 'performance of a patient', rather than of an intervention to a patient? Evaluate their performance in which respects, and for what purpose?

Perform comes from '*parfournir*' which, in old French, means 'to accomplish'. Who would find useful an evaluation of one patient or a group of patients' ability to accomplish self-care or adherence to a treatment or a healthy lifestyle? Who would find it useful to evaluate that before the patient does anything, or to evaluate their actual performance over time? Might different patients perform better in these respects? Would more educated patients perform better and would they need less support than others or would the reverse be true?

One method is to use the questionnaire developed by Hibbard et al. (2004) to assess the level of 'patient activation'. This is a term used to describe patients' replies to questions, some of which refer to actual performance, such as in maintaining lifestyle changes for health, and some of which cover attitudes and confidence, which may not be considered by some as 'performance'. Other examples are systems for evaluating patients' self-care for the side effects of cancer chemotherapy (Dodd 1982), for evaluating patients' performance in adhering to anti-depressant therapy (Cantrell et al. 2006) or more generally to assess self-efficacy (Lorig et al. 1989).

Three approaches can be used to evaluate a patient's performance in different respects: (1) to compare what they do with a standard (audit design), (2) with their own performance over time (single-case time-trend design) or (3) with other similar or different patients (comparative case design). Some patient risk assessment evaluation methods use audit designs to evaluate patients' performance in indulging in health-harming behaviours. Time-trend evaluation systems evaluate patient physiological performance over time to detect avoidable deterioration – some are computer-automated (McGaughey et al. 2007).

Conclusion

These example evaluations showed different designs applied to evaluate different interventions to patients. One – the doll example – was a low-cost, simple quasi-experimental evaluation. This certainly had its limitations but it did produce useful information for the evaluation user's decisions. The limitations to the certainty of the findings were carefully emphasized by the evaluators so as to reduce the chances of readers being misled by the apparent certainty which numbers give.

The comparative trial of the prescribing exercise example showed a more expensive and time-consuming design. These designs usually compare the intervention with a comparable one or none at all experienced by another group of patients. This helps to rule out influences on outcomes other than the intervention(s). Unusually, this design compared two similar interventions – the advantages of this were to show that similar effects could be observed in two different sites and the results are more likely to be generalizable than if only observed at one site.

The randomized controlled trial evaluation showed that this design can be used effectively to evaluate a complex intervention to patients – a package of services in the care transitions intervention. The internal validity was high, but so were the costs of the evaluation. There are questions about the generalizability of the results, about the details of the actual intervention used and about whether certain conditions would be needed elsewhere to implement it.

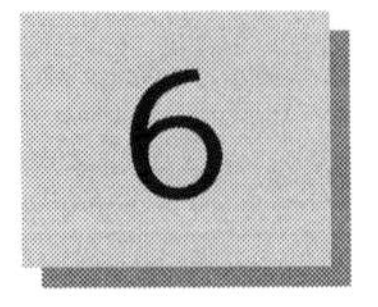

6 Evaluating interventions to professionals and performance evaluations

Introduction

This chapter summarizes three evaluations to show different designs for evaluating interventions to professionals. It shows how these designs answer different questions and illustrate how the designs that were outlined in Chapter 4 are applied. It shows the strengths and weaknesses of each design in giving the information needed by the evaluation users, within the constraints for the evaluation.

The chapter starts with an example of a simple mixed methods observational design to change the prescribing practices of physicians (Example 4). It then shows a quasi-experimental design to assess interventions to improve hand hygiene (Example 5). Example 6 is an observational process evaluation of intervention actions to enable providers to use methods to help patients stop smoking.

The chapter also notes different types of individual performance evaluation. Performance evaluation involves assessing dimensions of professionals' performance by comparing their performance in one or a number of respects.

Example 4 Mixed methods prospective observational evaluation of an intervention to change primary care physicians' behaviour

This evaluation (Nazareth et al. 2002) aimed to answer the question, 'Do educational outreach visits by pharmacists change primary care practitioners' (GPs) prescribing and what are the barriers and enablers of change?' A separate and related RCT assessed the effect of the intervention, and reported on changes in prescribing which were achieved (Freemantle et al. 2002), so it will be interesting to see if this implementation evaluation separately assesses outcomes or only refers to the outcomes discovered in the RCT.

The intervention evaluated community pharmacists visiting GPs in order to provide education about treatment recommendations for: angiotensin-converting enzyme inhibitors for the management of heart failure; aspirin for the secondary prevention of cardiovascular diseases; anti-depressant therapy for treating depression; and non-steroidal anti-inflammatory drugs for the management of osteoarthritis.

The design was a mixed methods and prospective observational evaluation. Each practice received an outreach visit for two topics and served as a control for the other two topics.

In this evaluation, the outcomes measured and discovered were: staged outcomes that included: (1) participation, attendance at an educational meeting; (2) pharmacists' assessment of the visits; (3) GPs' assessments of the visit (by questionnaire); and (4) change in prescribing of medications compared to guideline (which in fact uses the data reported in the RCT study (Freemantle et al. 2002)).

Results

Data on the pharmacists' assessment of the visits were given by their assessing the acceptability of the message to the GPs, their own overall performance, the rapport established with the doctors and the prediction of whether the doctors' prescribing practices would change. Nominal group interviews were used to assess the pharmacists' views of the interventions. Two group interviews were held: the first soon after the pharmacists had completed their initial visits and the second just before they had completed their last visit.

The details of the findings for each of the staged outcomes are given in the paper as well as the barriers discovered to changes in prescribing. As regards these changes, a 4 per cent change in prescribing for the anti-depressant guideline was observed and a 2 per cent change for the angiotensin-converting enzyme inhibitors guideline and 7 per cent for the aspirin guideline.

So, how certain can we be that these outcomes really come out of the intervention? The RCT study in fact answered the question: 'Does it work in terms of changing prescribing?' So we are not assessing this design for its ability to assess prescribing change. In contrast, this observational study was able to answer the questions: 'Why does it work?' and 'What helps and hinders?', as well as the reasons for different impacts on different types of prescribing.

How certain can we be about generalizability? As regards reproducing the intervention, the details provided would allow generalization, but whether the outcomes would be the same may depend more on the context in another setting. For example, financing for the drugs budget and incentives to reduce prescribing – these environmental aspects were not investigated in the study and not reported.

Strengths and weaknesses

Interestingly, this study alone could have given a less certain but useful answer at a lower cost than an RCT to the 'Does it change prescribing?' question, because the causal chain was mapped and the links between the staged outcomes could be established. The strengths were that it provided data which made it possible to discover the barriers to changes in prescribing and explain the different changes which were achieved. One weakness was that the sample may have been biased towards change-receptive GP practices: a number of GPs declined to take part.

Example 5 Interrupted time series evaluation of a hand hygiene intervention

Does a multifaceted hospital-wide intervention improve hand hygiene (HH) and reduce hospital-associated infection in patients? This was the question addressed in this example by Kirkland et al. (2012).

The interventions evaluated were carried out at different times, and included: (1) public statements by leadership; (2) measurement/feedback (monthly audits on all units published on an intranet site available to all staff, and reported to executive leadership, clinical leaders and board members); (3) increased hand sanitizer availability; (4) education/training using the internet and a certification programme for competency; and (5) marketing/communication with posters and screen savers, stories in medical centre publications and local news outlets, and direct communications with staff about expectations and progress towards goals.

The design was a three-year interrupted time series, with multiple sequential interventions, and one-year post-intervention follow-up (Figure 6.1).

Outcomes measured and discovered included: the intermediate outcome of implementation fidelity, by measuring the number of HH audits, the inventory of hand sanitizers utilized and the number of HH-related posters, screensavers and articles in internal publications. To assess staff exposure to the interventions,

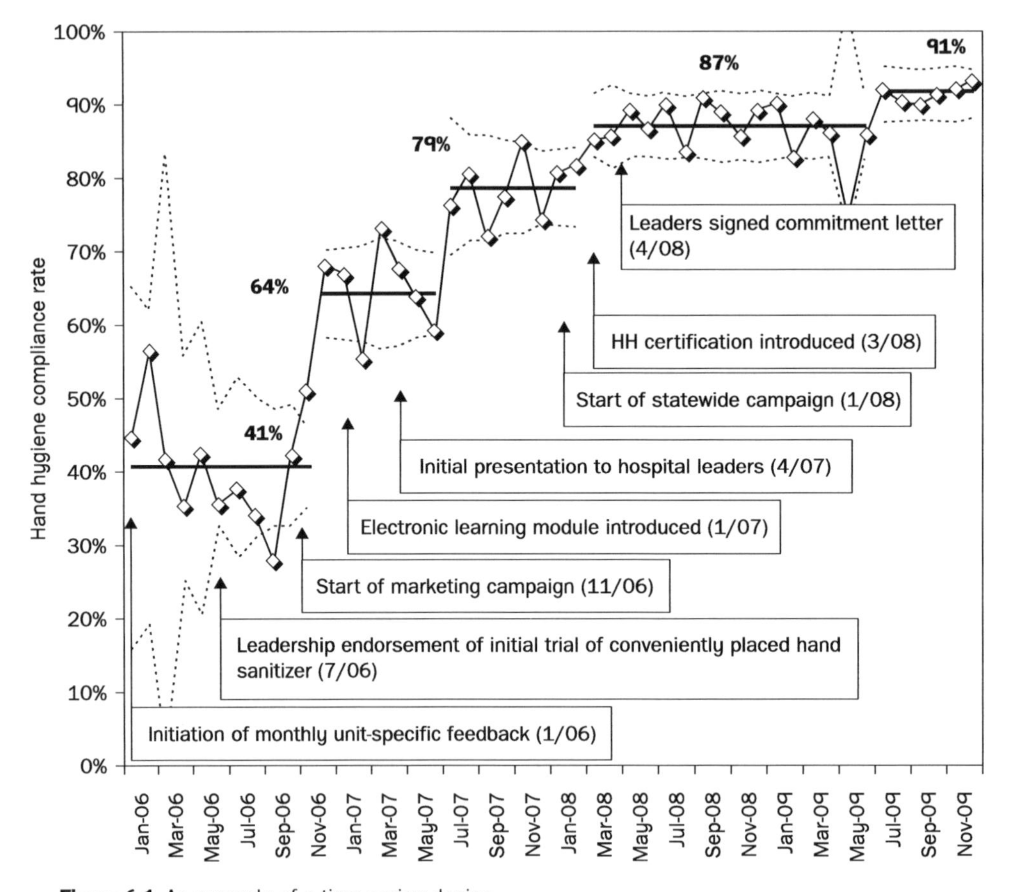

Figure 6.1 An example of a time series design

Source: Kirkland et al. (2012).

measures of the number of monthly visits to the report card website were used, as well as the completion rate for the electronic learning module and the number of staff who were certified 'competent' in HH.

Data were gathered about observed HH compliance (as a percentage): through direct covert observation by infection prevention staff (not blinded to the interventions), with training to ensure 90 per cent agreement in measurement during simultaneous observation periods. Monthly observations in all units counted HH 'opportunities' (before and after contact with patients or their immediate environments) and documented whether HH was performed (how was this done without staff being aware is not described in the report). Compliance percentage was defined as the number of times HH was performed by the total number of opportunities.

Rates of healthcare-associated infection per 1000 inpatient days were measured by a daily review of microbiology data, with a medical record review, and infection prevention staff applied standard definitions to identify all cases of bloodstream infection due to any organism, or clinical infection at any site due to Staphylococcus aureus and Clostridium difficile infection.

Did it work?

The evaluation reported three sets of results: (1) quite high intervention fidelity; (2) improved HH compliance; and (3) associations of the presence of interventions with a decline in infection rates, suggesting that interventions did contribute to reduce infections although the amount each contributed is not clear. Compliance rates per units are shown in Figure 6.2.

Physician HH rates, using statistical process control analysis, are shown in Figure 6.3, and infections attributable to OR/1000 surgical cases are shown in Figure 6.4.

Figure 6.5 shows the infections associated with inpatient and outpatient care/1000 inpatient days and Figure 6.6 is a scatter plot of monthly healthcare-associated infection index rates and hand hygiene compliance rates.

Strengths and weaknesses

As regards attribution confidence, one strength was the assessment of stages in the causal chain made possible by the time series design, which increased certainty that the outcomes were due to the intervention: the stages assessed were: (1) extent of implementation; (2) HH compliance; and (3) infection rates. Another strength was the actions taken to select and collect a few key measures, their validity for the question, and the accuracy of the data collected on (1), (2) and (3). These strengths are not necessarily intrinsic to the type of design (other observational designs include these elements), but show best practice in using this type of design.

The certainty of attribution may be less because of the observation method, which may be an intervention in its own right: some staff must have known about monthly 'direct covert observation', so the intervention is not just feedback of data but also either awareness of being observed or knowing an observer is present. Also a

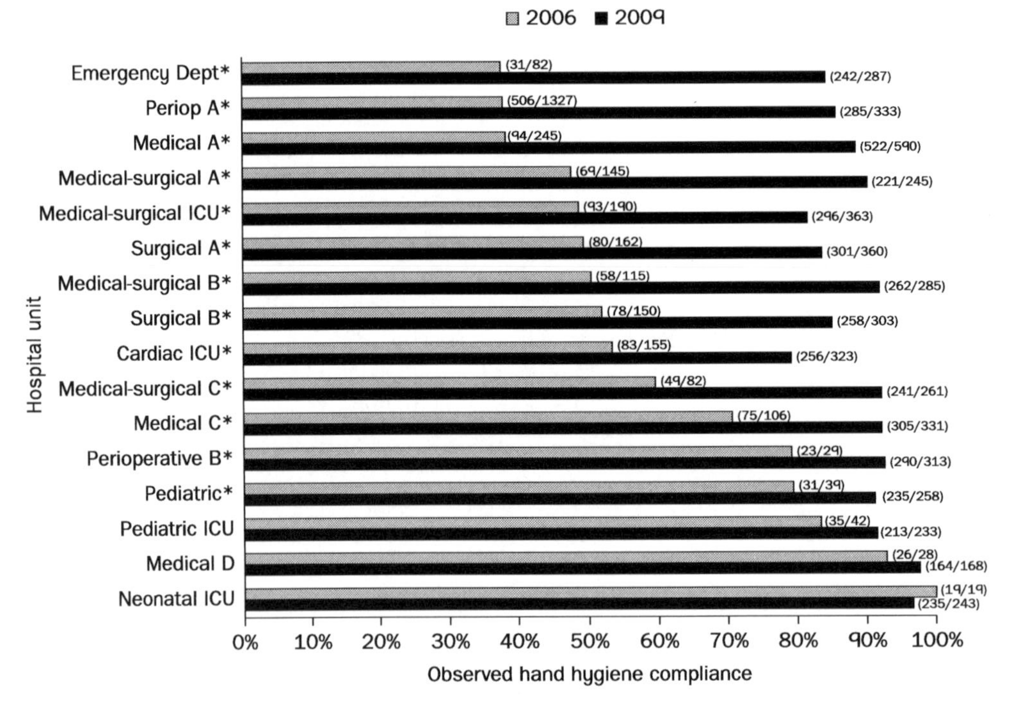

Figure 6.2 Compliance rates of HH per unit

Source: Kirkland et al. (2012).

simultaneous statewide campaign – the 'High Five for a Healthy NH' – may have contributed to the results.

Could others apply the same intervention and get the same results? The reproducibility of the intervention may be questionable because of the high cost. Timely feedback as an essential part of many CSIs and both process (compliance) and outcome data (infections) are collected for credibility. However, the cost of this, especially monthly observations of all units, may be too high for many hospitals, so these costs may make generalizability difficult without data on savings and a return on investment assessment.

Other strengths and weaknesses of the design in this example

Sustained hand hygiene compliance is one of the most difficult changes to achieve and requires a CSI which includes an infrastructure and systems to sustain it (the latter was not described in the study). One strength was the assessment of stages in the causal chain noted above to increase the confidence of attribution. Also, the study used a 'tracer condition' less sensitive to hand hygiene – infections attributed to the operating room – as a comparison: that this rose at the same time as the other data increases certainty that these were due to the intervention.

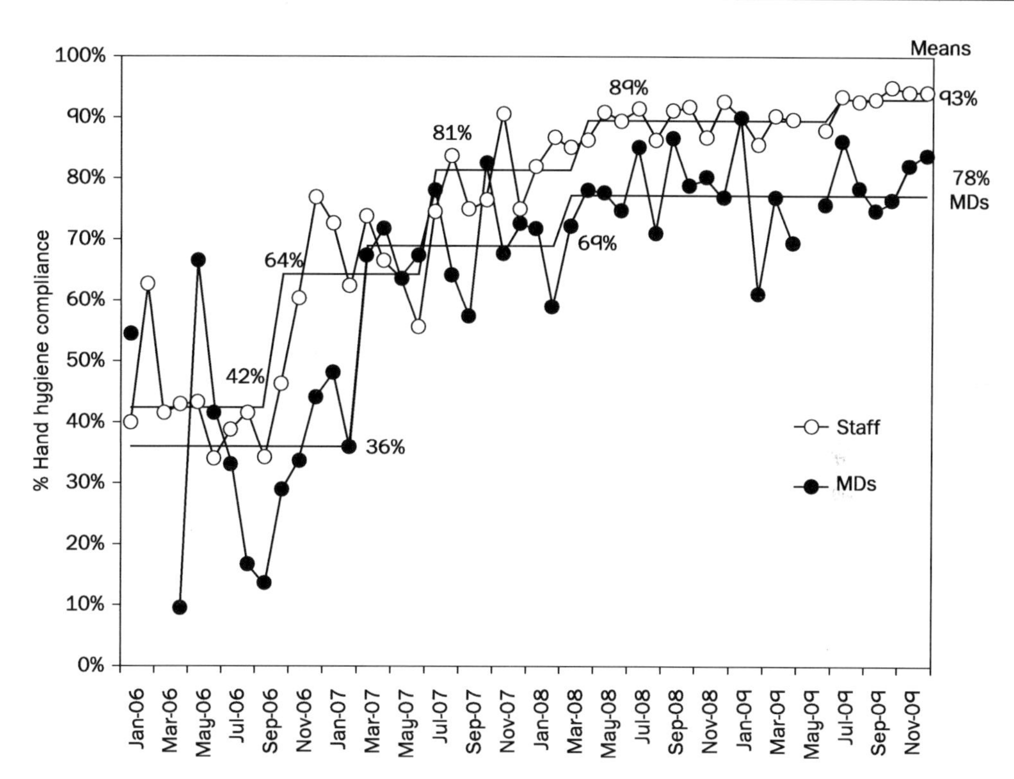

Figure 6.3 Physician HH compliance rates

Source: Kirkland et al. (2012).

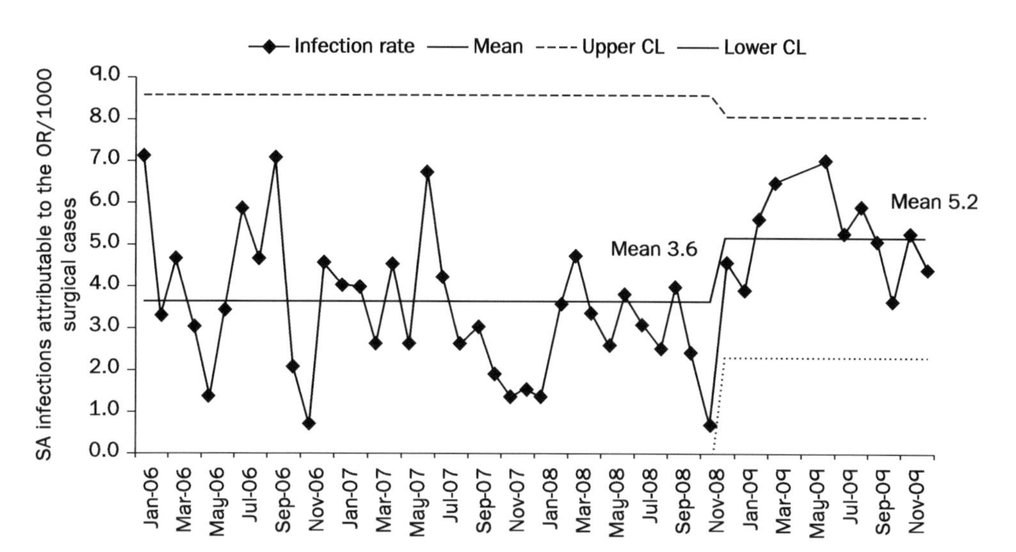

Figure 6.4 Infections attributable to OR/1000 surgical cases

Source: Kirkland et al. (2012).

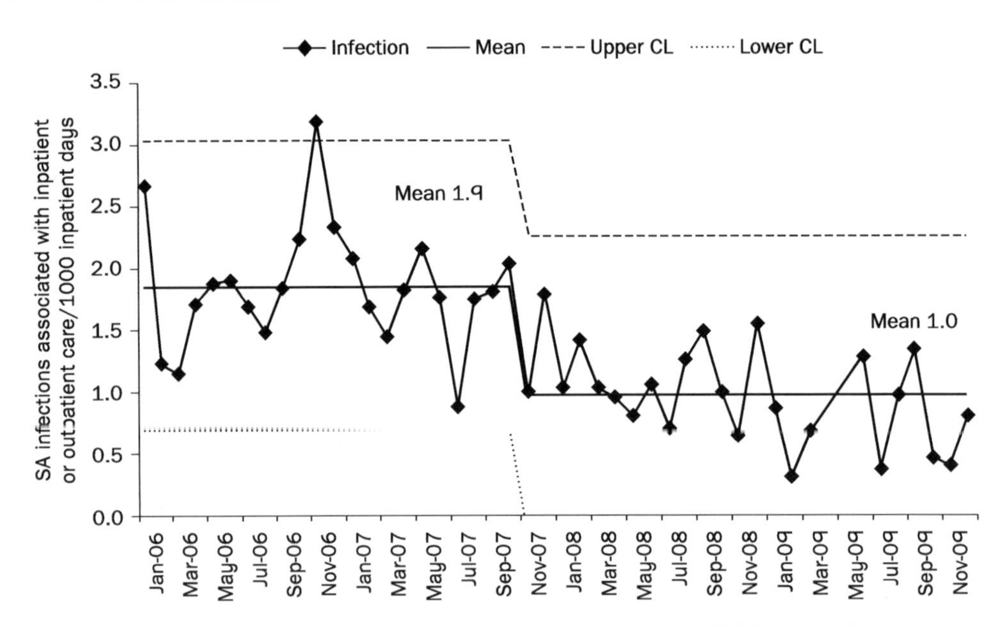

Figure 6.5 Infections associated with inpatient and outpatient care/1000 inpatient days

Source: Kirkland et al. (2012).

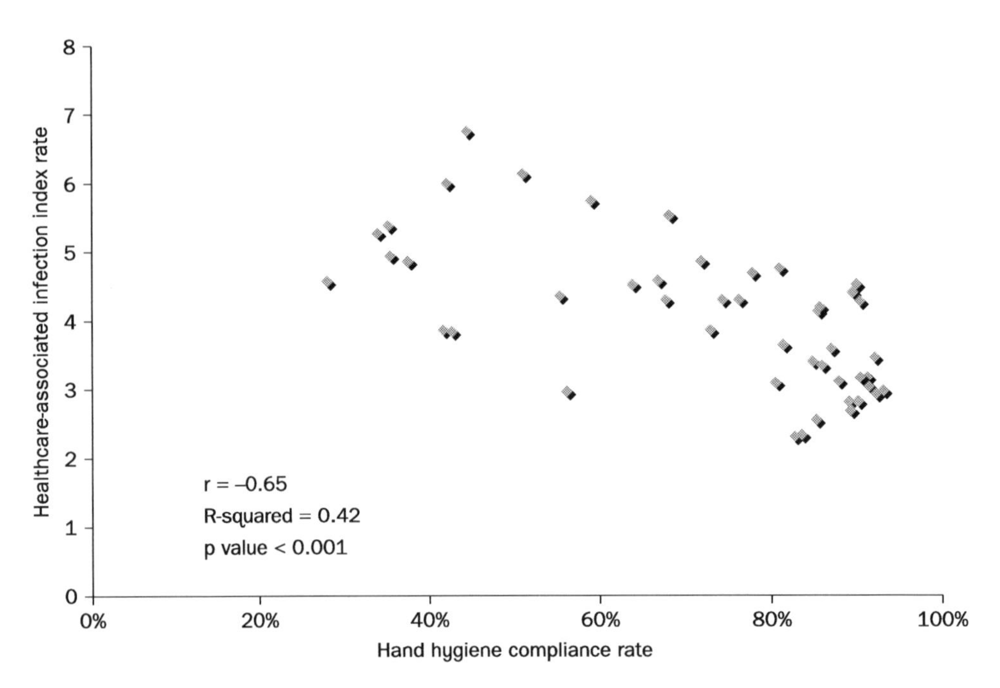

Figure 6.6 Monthly healthcare-associated infection index rates and hand hygiene compliance rates

The design was able to accommodate the evolution of the programme. But it should be noted that it did not give exact details of the interventions introduced or intensified over the three years. This does not allow us to assess exactly which interventions had more of an impact than others, or how much the results depended on a whole programme and a synergy between the components or the staging of the components.

Another strength of the study, but not intrinsic to this design, was the use of process control charts. These helped to decide if the change was random or due to a special cause, and also to monitor the impact of the phased introduction of the interventions.

As with other studies of this type, it is the differences between subjects or units that are of interest: although the design was able to show this, it could not explain the differences. This is a limitation on the study. An additional retrospective study could have been made, using another design and could have used insights of the compliance observers to build a theory.

Example 6 Process evaluation of an intervention to promote smoking cessation

This evaluation aimed to answer the question 'How was the "Quit Together" intervention implemented to improve smoking cessation and relapse prevention among low-income pregnant and postpartum women who receive care at community health centers (CHCs)?' (Zapka et al. 2004). This was a US-based intervention.

The evaluation report described the intervention evaluated as a theory- and evidence-based intervention with three components: (1) a provider-delivered smoking intervention, with providers trained to deliver guideline-based, tailored counselling at all visits; (2) prompts to providers, using an office practice-management system tailored to each clinic (to screen for smoking status, deliver the intervention, document the encounter, distribute materials, and arrange follow-up for patients); and (3) processes to help systematic communication and documentation linkages between clinics to promote consistency and continuity of the smoking cessation strategies for women.

The design was a process evaluation of implementation participation and interactions (Figure 6.7). Smoking cessation services at the six comparison 'usual care' sites were clinical interventions without protocols. A separate controlled trial was carried out to assess the outcome.

Outcomes measured and discovered

Process data were collected using eight methods:

1 *Organizational assessment (OA) reports.* Collected from key informant interviews about programme/clinic flow, structure, and process linkages among the clinics and key players. The interviews were analysed to identify potential barriers and facilitators to integration of the intervention into each clinic of each SI health centre's operations.

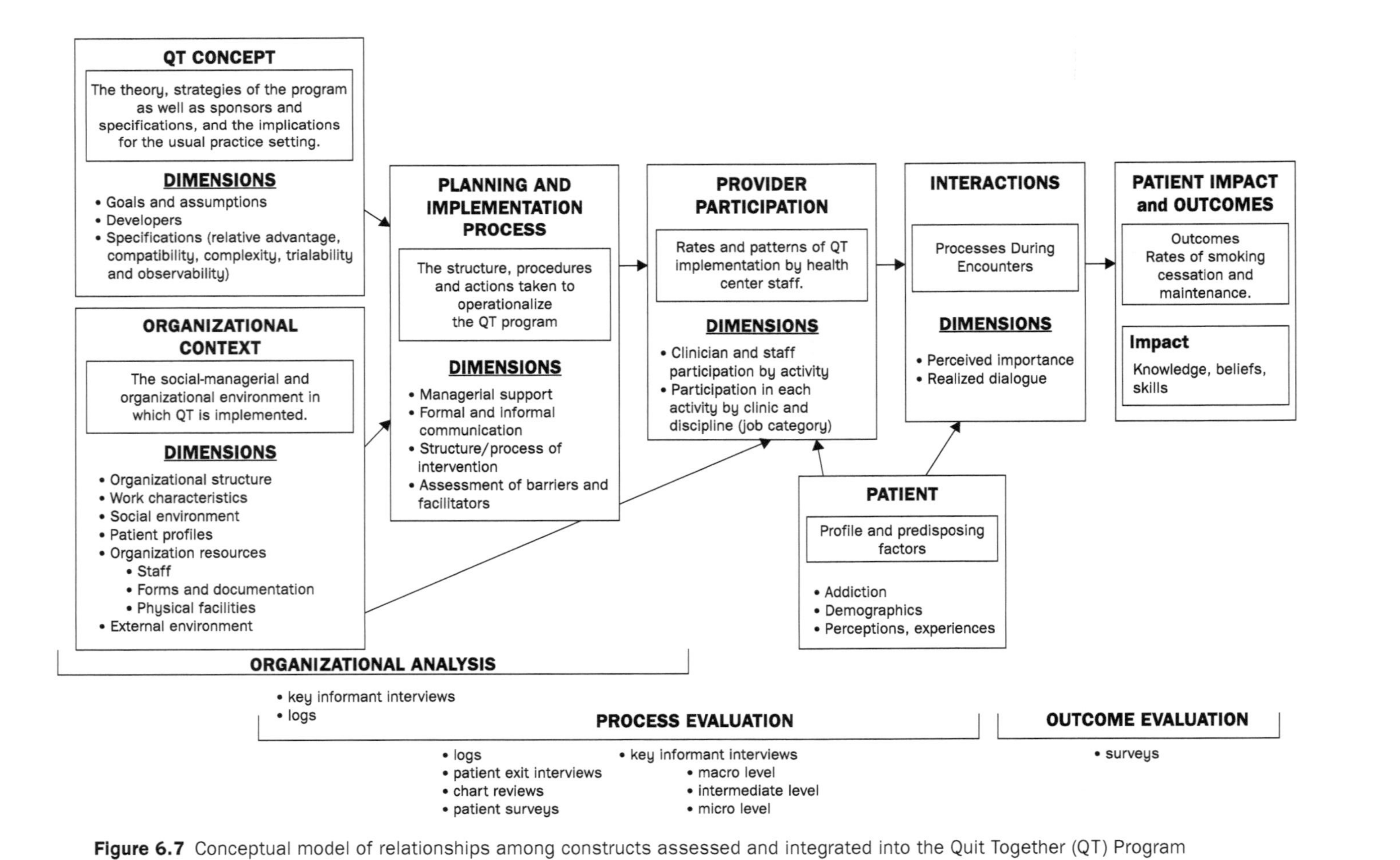

Figure 6.7 Conceptual model of relationships among constructs assessed and integrated into the Quit Together (QT) Program

2 *Contact logs.* A semi-structured form to record the intervention coordinator's meetings with key personnel at each SI clinic, to track the expectations from each meeting and whether follow-up occurred. (It was reported that, from this, the coordinator 'identified the underlying problem of a power struggle between two key individuals. She then tailored her actions to move the project forward'.)
3 *Meeting notes.* For meetings of the programme boards, clinic work groups, and individual personnel key to the project, recording the type of meeting, the participants, the agenda, the issues discussed and the decisions made.
4 *Training records.* A Microsoft Access database was developed to track all SI providers trained.
5 *Key informant interviews (KIIs).* Follow-up interviews halfway and at the end of the trial.
6 *Patient exit interviews (PEI).* After every WI clinic nutrition appointment.
7 *Patient report of exposure in periodic surveys.* At the final prenatal interview, questions prompted the patient to think about her most recent visit to the Obstetrics clinic. At the postpartum interviews, questions asked the patient to confirm implementation of the intervention protocol steps at her most recent paediatric visit.
8 *Medical record reviews.* Clinic staff at SI sites (1) placed a cue on each woman's record ('chart') to remind providers to intervene for smoking, and (2) placed guidance in the chart to help providers record what they had done. A random sample of charts of women eligible for the study was examined to confirm the presence of the cue and guidance in the record and completeness of documentation (Figure 6.8).

The main findings were about challenges to implementation of the Quit Together strategy, which explained programme implementation failure, specifically concerning organizational context, planning and implementation.

As regards confidence about and generalizability of the outcomes: this process evaluation triangulated and compared data from the KII, logs, and chart reviews were examined across clinic types (OB, PED, and WIC) for each site, across sites for each clinic type and across intervention condition (SI vs. UC) using the 'Constant comparison method' (Lincoln and Guba, 1985). These methods increased the certainty about the findings.

The strengths of the design were that relevant data from the PEIs and periodic patient surveys also were reviewed. Observations were reported according to the domains identified in the pre-study theory of the intervention bearing in mind three types of potential failure: theory, programme implementation, and measurement failure. Translating the contextual factors into lessons for practitioners was conducted considering these three areas. This design was able to examine context factors affecting complex programmes of this type and show the 'lessons learned' about barriers and approaches needed for implementation in similar programmes.

Summary of Observations
(Data Source in Parentheses)

The QT Concept

Goals and Assumptions

The concept of the intervention was met with enthusiasm at all levels of the organization. Commitment to tobacco treatment as an important issue facilitated moving forward with the trial.

The assumption of three key components (provider intervention, office management, and clinic linkages) was embraced.

Developers

Impetus came from the academic partners. A highly skilled intervention director was initially able to engage administrators and clinicians in refining the intervention to best fit their needs.

Specifications

The continuum of care for pregnant and postpartum women envisioned by academic and service partners proved inaccurate (NA , CL, M). The reality of relative autonomy of clinic operations meant changes resulting in real continuity could not be implemented.

Cooperation across clinics within community health centers (CHCs] was more difficult than anticipated. This was exacerbated at some sites by the complexity of medical records systems (NA, CL, M). Anticipated linkages were either not implemented or not sustained.

Nature of Change

Supplemental Food Program for Women, Infants, and Children (WIC) was not well enough integrated into the health care mission and culture of CHCs (CL). Cross-clinic communication and documentation were initially expected and viewed as beneficial.

Individual clinicians perceive smoking as important, however, special passion is needed over time. The three-component approach would hopefully build commitment.

The Organizational Context

Organizational Structure

Five of the six participating health centers underwent either a merger or financial restructuring during the grant period, resulting in a high degree of turmoil and chaos for each institution (NA, KII, M). Leadership and staff were distracted. Meetings were hard to schedule. Relationship building was difficult. Constant change meant difficulty not only implementing but institutionalizing change.

Several clinics experienced changes to their physical space, either moves or renovations (KII, M). The intervention became lower priority when execution of regular duties was made more difficult because of physical space issues.

Individuals key to project implementation and/or facilitation of research tasks were difficult to identify (NA CL). Lack of sufficient buy-in from key players led to passive neglect or, less uncommonly, active resistance. The merger at one site brought new key individuals identification of whom was a low priority for providers involved with the intervention.

Few perinatal work groups or committees existed prior to intervention implementation, resulting in little formal communication among clinics (NA, KII). The program board concept was implemented with mixed results. The approach for each clinic of each site had to be highly tailored to organizational structure.

Some clinics lacked strong leadership for the intervention (CL, M). Intervention implementation was often delayed, and full integration of the intervention into the organization was not always achieved.

Decision-making authority regarding the intervention was often unclear (CL, M). Critical decisions were delayed as the intervention coordinator sought to determine who had authority for a given aspect.

Difficulties resulting from a merger cut across an entire institution and distracted staff attention from the study. Occasional struggles between different types of clinicians or management within some clinics also contributed (M).

High staff turnover (16% to 41%) occurred throughout the study (T). The intervention director continually engaged in new relationship building and training.

The high level of patient scheduling and rescheduling was not anticipated in planning the research.

Social Environment

Staff morale was affected by organizational chaos (M) The intervention director found it difficult to build enthusiasm for the intervention or establish it as a priority for the staff individually.

Cooperation within and across clinics crucial for such a complex intervention was not established (CL, M).

External Environment

The Massachusetts Tobacco Control Program (MTCP) was viewed as a positive force (M). MTCP initially presented a historical threat to internal validity, as its programs prompted activity in usual care (UC) sites.

The Planning and Implementation Process

Buy-in from advisory boards varied across sites. Low buy-in resulted in the impression that the intervention director, rather than the CHC staff, was ultimately accountable (M). Approach needs to be highly flexible and tailored for each unit (site) and subunit (clinic). Strong leadership is needed for cross-clinic communication.

Every step took much longer than anticipated. The research timeline did not allow sufficient time for all phases (M, KII).

Figure 6.8 Summary of observations

Note: Data sources in parentheses.

Source: Zapka et al. (2004).

Evaluating individual professional performance

Your performance, as a physician, declines the older you get. This is what one study concluded after reviewing evaluations of physician performance. It also found many evaluations reported decreasing performance with increasing experience, at least for some outcomes (Choudhry et al. 2005).

Have you undergone a 'performance appraisal'? Many of us have self-assessed, or been part of a peer assessment process, or had our manager carry out a periodic performance assessment, usually with our participation. These are all evaluations of individual performance for different purposes and using different methods.

For many professionals, this is a controversial subject, even for the purposes of self-improvement. And especially if used by a physician's employing or paying organization, or for pay-for-performance schemes. In the UK, various scandals have prompted much discussion and a number of different systems such as a general medical practioner 'revalidation' process (RCGP 2013). Individual performance assessment systems are not going away, but will increase: the issue is to develop or use the best evaluation method for the purpose.

Are they effective for their purpose? Is the cost worth the changes they may influence? These are two questions asked of performance assessment interventions. However, in this section, we note only the designs and methods used for evaluating individual performance and do not address methods for evaluating whether they are effective as interventions on their own or used with other interventions such as payment.

Comparing one person's performance to their performance last month, or last year, is one common approach to performance evaluation. Another is comparing their performance to a 'similar person'. Both approaches compare specific aspects of performance in order to improve performance. Most systems for individual performance improvement use these evaluations to then decide actions and interventions which would help the professional improve.

One approach is to use already collected indicators. Another is to collect data directly for the evaluation, if no suitable already collected indicators can be used. An example of the former is the evaluation system used by Vanderbilt Medical Center in the USA, which draws on patient complaints and malpractice claims data which provide one way to evaluate one aspect of physician performance (Hickson and Pichert 2007). More details and guidance can be found at Landon et al. (2003).

Conclusion

Different interventions for professionals exist for different purposes. Few have been evaluated, though we do know a fair bit about which are effective in enabling professionals to follow guidelines (Grimshaw et al. 2004). The chapter considered an example of a simple mixed methods observational design to change physicians' prescribing practice. It then showed a quasi-experimental design to assess interventions to improve hand hygiene. The third shows an observational process evaluation of an intervention to enable providers to use methods to help patients stop smoking. The chapter also noted different types of individual performance evaluation. The chapter showed that there are strengths and weaknesses to the designs which have been used to evaluate this type of intervention, depending on the purpose of the evaluation and the resources available for it.

Evaluating interventions to health services and performance

Introduction

Many interventions to health services involve training to change what individual providers do in their daily work. Chapter 6 looked at interventions to individual providers: why do we need a separate chapter now to look at interventions to health services? Surely these are to change the people who work on these services in some way? Why might we need distinctly different methods for evaluating interventions to health services as organizations, to those used to evaluate interventions to individuals? This introduction first answers these questions, before outlining the examples and evaluation methods discussed later in the chapter.

A patient safety programme for a hospital is an intervention to one type of health service. The programme uses activities to train providers and to change procedures and arrangements to reduce risks and adverse events to patients. A hospital, like a primary care centre, a clinic or department of public health, is a service organization. It organizes the work of many individuals to provide services through procedures and uses systems to support and coordinate them. But these explicit arrangements are the 'tip of the iceberg': the main way in which we regularize our working together to get so much done is through the informal rules and norms, some of which is hinted at by the abused term 'culture'.

This way of understanding health services as subjects of the intervention is important to how we use evaluation designs to evaluate the intervention. Chapter 1 noted that every evaluation carries with it a conception of the subject which the intervention is seeking to change. Both interventions and evaluations involve assumptions about the subjects of the intervention: is the intervention to a machine or a biological process, or to a conscious human subject, or to a work organization, or to a residential community?

The point is that the subject of the interventions in this chapter are social entities rather than a collection of individual human beings. The hospital is not the sum total of all the individuals' activities: it is something beyond and above this. Interventions to change organizational performance, but which only intervene on individuals, inevitably fail because the social features and systems that influence individuals at work are untouched.

An intervention to a working organization is different from an intervention to an individual and evaluations need to bear this in mind. Evaluations of interventions to service organizations need to describe and assess any changes beyond those which are made directly to individuals, such as training. They need also to assess whether changes are made to procedures, systems and culture and to the conditions under which individuals work, whether or not these were part of the intervention.

In this chapter, we consider interventions to healthcare services rather than other health services, such as a public health department. The principles for evaluating interventions to other types of service in the health sector are the same.

The chapter summarizes three evaluations to show how different designs are applied to evaluate interventions to health services: first, an intervention to intensive care units (Example 7), then a large-scale safety programme intervening on a number of hospitals (Example 8), then an intervention to health services to enable them to make and use electronic summaries of electronic medical records (EMRs) (Example 9).

These are all interventions to services. At the end, the chapter also considers performance evaluations of health services. These evaluate the performance of the service in relation to defined criteria and where there is no specific intervention to the service being evaluated. Rather, the intervention is the service itself, which intervenes to patients, and the service performance in terms of its impact on the patient population is evaluated, as well as its performance in other respects.

The chapter also shows the strengths and weaknesses of each design in giving the information needed by the evaluation users within the constraints for the evaluation.

Example 7 Pragmatic cluster RCT of a multi-component intervention to 15 intensive care units

In the USA, intensive care units in smaller 'community hospitals' do not have as many resources as those in larger academic medical centers (AMCs). Will interventions which work in AMCs also be successful in such services? This evaluation aimed to answer the question: does a complex intervention to community-based critical care units (ICUs) increase adherence to six quality activities, each of which have been documented to improve patient outcomes (Scales et al. 2011)? Essentially, this was an evaluation of an education and support programme for ICUs, delivered on the internet, with other related components.

One question to the reader is, should the evaluation be limited to finding out if the intervention led to personnel following the quality activities? Or should it also evaluate relevant outcomes for patients – outcomes which are believed to occur if these quality activities are undertaken? The answer might be 'no', if the question was defined after discussion with the users about what they wanted from the evaluation – which may have been only to find out if these quality activities were being carried out. Still, we might wonder how good the evidence is that these quality activities really do improve patient outcomes and how others had evaluated this.

Another related question, given that this evaluation was not about whether the quality activities improve patient outcomes, is whether this evaluation is an implementation evaluation. If it is only to evaluate the effectiveness of an intervention to increase the use of these quality activities, then it would appear to be an evaluation of a particular implementation strategy. The following summarizes the evaluation and returns to these questions.

The intervention which was evaluated was implemented sequentially and included education, dissemination of guidance and procedures, and audit and feedback, transferred through an interactive telecommunication strategy (video conference-based forum). The subjects (targets) of the intervention were personnel in 15 different ICUs in 15 different community hospitals in the USA (Table 7.1).

Table 7.1 Components of the Quality Improvement Intervention

Intervention	Description
Educational outreach	Monthly videoconference with study coordinators to discuss progress and implementation strategies
	Videoconferenced educational sessions provided by content experts for each evidence-based care practice; available for later viewing on Web site
	Development of a bibliography of evidence-based literature supporting each targeted care practice
	Summary of guidelines into easy-to-read bulletins
	Support of local champions in presenting educational sessions
Reminders and other tools	Promotional items (posters, bulletins, lapels, pens, stamps, pocket cards)
	Preprinted order sets
	Checklists
Audit and feedback	Daily audit of process-of-care indicators
	Monthly reports of performance measures to each ICU
	Each ICU's performance compared anonymously to peer ICUs

Source: Scales et al. (2011).

The design

The design chosen was a pragmatic cluster randomized controlled trial (RCT). In this design, both an 'experimental' group (n = seven ICUs) and the 'control group' (n = eight ICUs) received the intervention. But sequencing was used so that, over four months, a different care practice was intended for the experimental group to that intended for the control group ICUs (Figure 7.1). Put another way, this means during each four-month phase of the trial, each group of ICUs received one active behaviour change intervention targeting one care practice and simultaneously acted as a control group for the other group of ICUs that received the active behaviour change intervention targeting a different care practice. This avoided randomizing a group of ICUs to no intervention, which, the researchers say, 'could have been demoralizing'.

Different outcomes were measured and discovered. The measures were selected to assess whether the six activities thought to improve patient outcomes changed as a

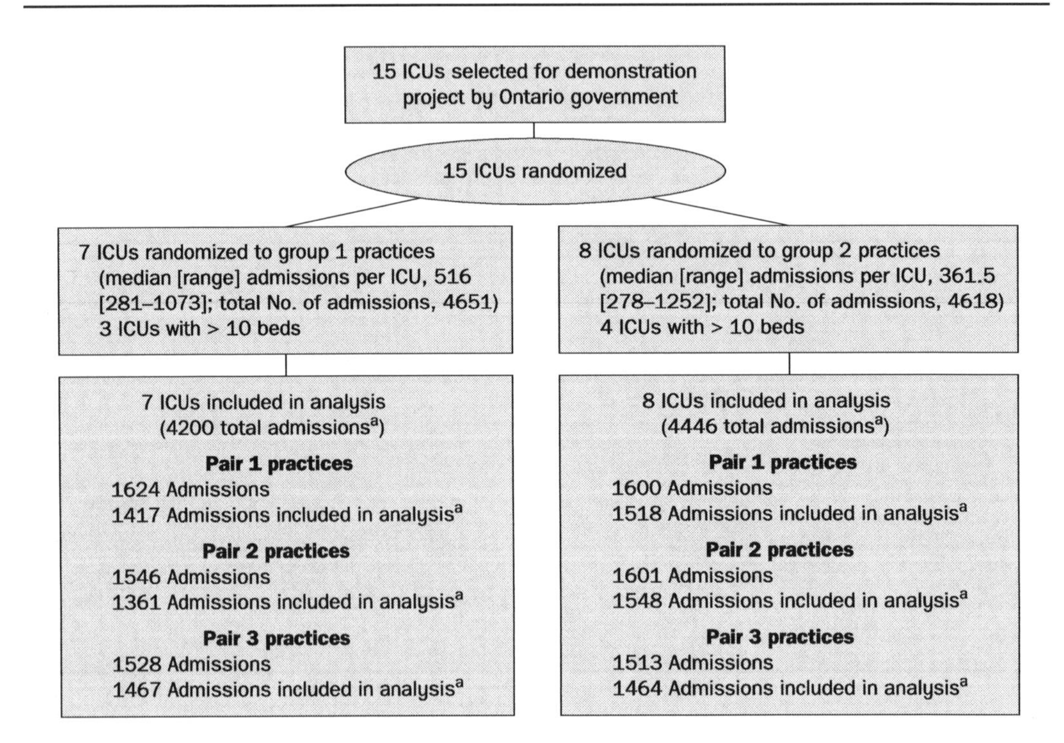

Figure 7.1 Selection and allocation of 15 ICUs for demonstration project
Source: Scales et al. (2011).

result of the intervention, and by how much. The activities included those: (1) to prevent ventilator-associated pneumonia (VAP); (2) to increase prophylaxis for deep venous thrombosis (DVT); (3) to increase daily spontaneous breathing trials; (4) to prevent catheter-related bloodstream infections (CRBIs); (5) to increase early enteral feeding; and (6) to prevent pressure ulcers.

Table 7.2 from the report shows a number of process of care indicators and measures which were collected from different data sources, using different data collection methods.

Each participating ICU selected a data collector (a nurse or a ward clerk not providing patient care), who received data collection training from the central trial coordinating office. To record data, they used handheld wireless electronic devices that connected to a central database via a local server. The measure definition was the presence of one process of care indicator and no contraindications to receiving the practice. Data were collected once daily.

The findings were that, overall, patients in ICUs receiving active intervention were more likely to receive the targeted care practice than those in the contemporaneous control ICUs receiving an active intervention to a different practice. There were, however, significant differences between how much each care practice was increased compared to the 'control'. This difference is most clear in the figures reporting change in the use of practices between experimental and control ICUs (Figure 7.2).

Table 7.2 Process of care indicators for each targeted care practice

Care Practice	Process-of-Care Indicators	Main Measurement	Other Measurements
Prevention of ventilator-associated pneumonia	Semirecumbent positioning Orotracheal intubation	No. of eligible patient-days with head of bed ≥30°	No. of eligible patient-days associated with orotracheal (vs nasotracheal) intubation
Prophylaxis against deep vein thrombosis	Administration of anticoagulant prophylaxis Use of antiembolic stockings if anticoagulant prophylaxis contraindicated	No. of eligible patients receiving appropriate anticoagulant prophylaxis within 48 h	No. of eligible patient-days associated with receipt of anticoagulant prophylaxis Ineligible days associated with use of antiembolic stockings
Daily spontaneous breathing trials	Spontaneous breathing trial or extubation within previous 24 h	No. of eligible patient-days on which spontaneous breathing trial (or extubation) was performed	
Prevention of catheter-related bloodstream infections	7-Point checklist for sterile insertion completed Fulfillment of all 7 criteria listed on checklist Anatomical site of catheter insertion	No. of central venous catheters inserted using all 7 criteria on checklist	No. of central venous catheters inserted at the subclavian site (vs jugular or femoral sites)
Early enteral feeding	Initiation of enteral feeds within 48 h of ICU admission	No. of eligible patients receiving early enteral feeding within 48 h of ICU admission	No. of eligible patients achieving 50% of their target caloric goal via the enteral route by 72 h
Decubitus ulcer prevention	Completion of the Braden index at least daily	No. of patient-days with Braden index completed	

Source: Scales et al. (2011).

These figures compare how much the intervention appears to have increased the use of the quality practice of the risk assessment for decubitus ulcer, compared to the insignificant increase in the practice of increased prophylaxis for deep venous thrombosis (DVT). The authors suggest that some care practices were more amenable to improvement through this type of intervention than others.

As regards certainty about and generalizability of the outcomes, the randomization and parallel switching of the interventions in the two groups did reduce the number of other explanations for the outcomes. But this does require complex data collection and analysis. An observational study would not have been able to exclude temporal change as an explanation for the findings in the same way. The study also used a 'decay-monitoring period' to assess if the improvements persisted and used interviews with participants to discover possible ways in which the intervention had its effect and what helped and hindered.

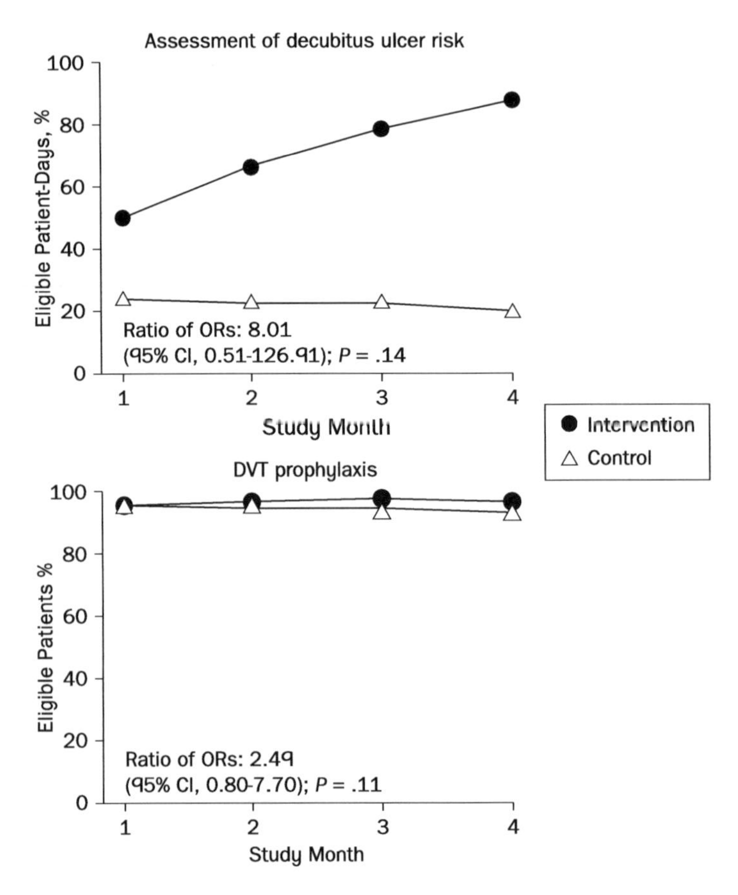

Figure 7.2 Change in the use of practices between experimental and control ICUs
Source: Scales et al. (2011).

As regards repeating the intervention, the time resources and effort to implement the trial were largely provided by the research and these resources may not be available elsewhere.

What are the strengths and weaknesses of the design in this example? As regards the outcome measures, those chosen are indicators which are thought to correlate with patient outcomes, but the evidence of this correlation could be contested. It is a long and fragile causal chain from carrying out a pressure ulcer risk assessment to reductions in pressure ulcer incidence. Following the care practice – risk assessment – cannot be said with certainty to then result in better patient outcomes, and this criticism applies to many of the other five 'quality practices'. Even though there were over 9000 ICU admissions, this was not a large enough sample size to find differences in patient outcomes. A trial to do this would be too large and expensive to be feasible, and requiring patient-level outcomes would have slowed down the study.

A strength of the design is the useful evidence it provided about how the intervention appears to have significantly improved three care practices (for VAP positioning, changes to catheter practices, and pressure ulcer risk assessment) but had little impact on three others (DVT prophylaxis, daily SBT and early enteral nutrition).

This study deployed its data collection resources to collect a range of measures from each ICU. The disadvantage of this is there is not much research time and resources available to assess the validity and comparability of the data, so there may be questions about data accuracy. The report notes a site inspection and audit of data collection at each ICU during the trial, but no further details are given. The primary outcome (summary ratio of odds ratios) is complicated to compute and understand, but is appropriate for the research question. Overall, we note that cluster randomized trials are complex and not easy to carry out successfully.

Example 8 Mixed methods, prospective, observational evaluation of a large-scale safety programme

This second discussion of design is of the value in four hospitals taking part in a programme in the UK called Safer Patients Initiative' (SPI) (Benning et al. 2011). The question was: 'What are the effects of the first phase of a multi-component intervention on four participating hospitals, each in different countries in the UK?' This was an organizational intervention similar to the US IHI 100,000 lives campaign, using quality improvement breakthrough methods (Berwick et al. 2006). These included interventions to improve specific care processes in certain clinical specialties and to promote organizational and cultural change. The design was a mixed method before and after evaluation, with five sub-studies (Figure 7.3). There were four intervention hospitals compared to 18 'control' hospitals.

Outcomes measured and discovered

The UK National Health Service conducts regular staff survey questionnaires. This was used to provide data at two time points about staff morale, attitudes, and aspects of 'culture' that might be affected by the generic strengthening of organizational systems that the SPI aimed to achieve.

For the qualitative study, one researcher undertook three rounds of data collection. Between April and September 2006, she visited one medical ward in each of the four hospitals for one week for 150 hours of ethnographic observations and conducted 47 interviews with different types of ward staff, focusing on general issues relating to patient safety. Medical case notes were reviewed for much of the other data (Table 7.3).

Findings

The findings were that, overall, the introduction of the first phase of the SPI evaluated in these hospitals was associated with improvements in one of the types of clinical process studied (monitoring of vital signs) and in one measure of staff perceptions of organizational climate. Few data were found indicating any additional effect of this part of the SPI on other objectives of the SPI, or from other measures of generic organizational strengthening (Figure 7.4).

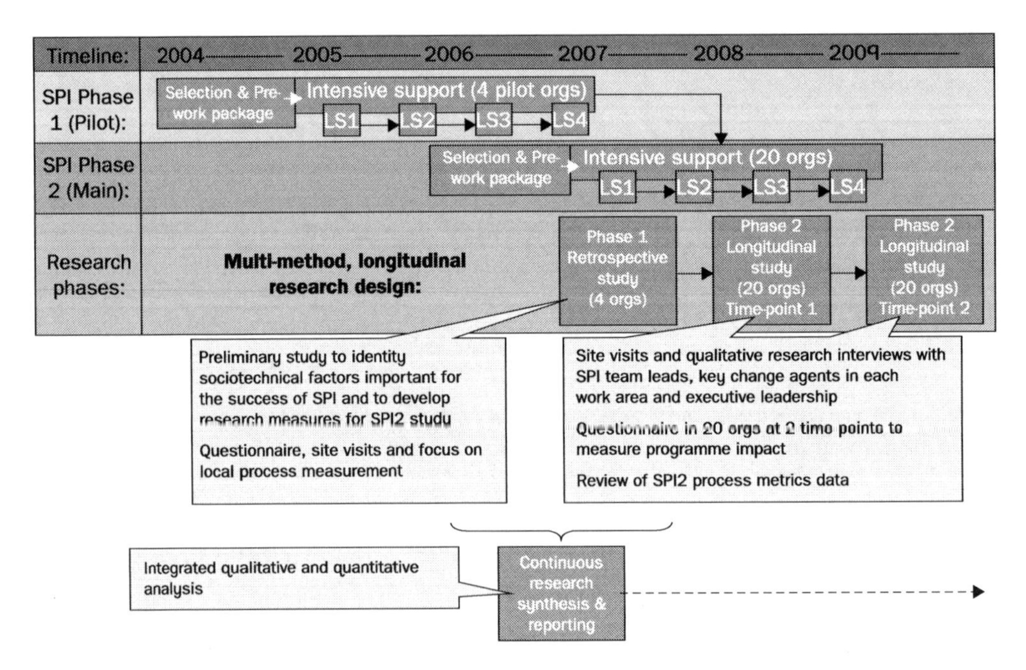

Figure 7.3 Multi-method longitudinal research design for the SPI evaluation

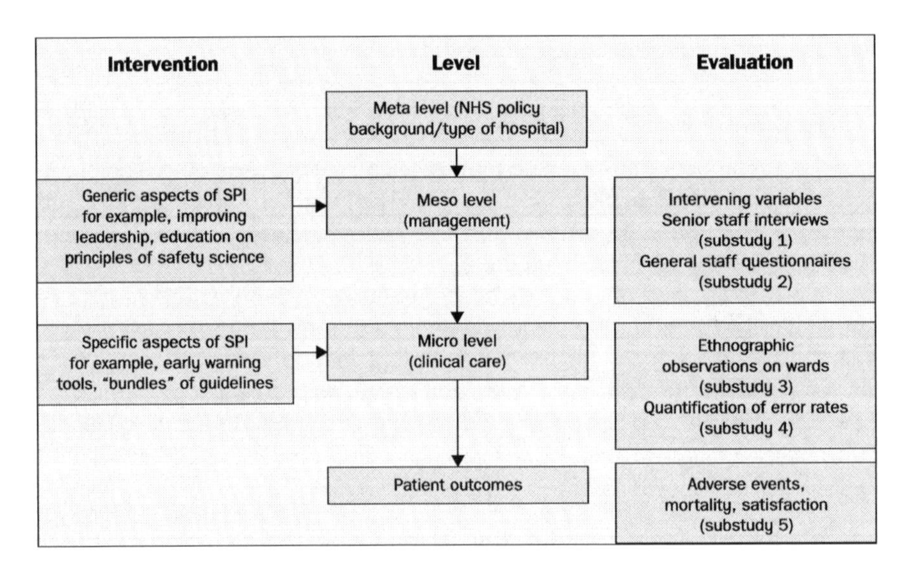

Figure 7.4 Relationship between the intervention, the levels and the evaluation in the SPI study
Source: Benning et al. (2011).

Table 7.3 Summary of sub-studies comprising evaluation of phase one of Safer Patients Initiative (SPI1)

Substudy and topic	Data source	Location	Unit of analysis (quantitative studies)
Interviews with senior staff			
Impact of SPI at senior management level	Semistructured interviews with senior hospital staff	SPI1 hospitals	NA
Staff survey			
Staff morale, culture, and opinion	Questionnaire as used in NHS National Staff Survey	Control and SPI1 hospitals	Staff member
Qualitative study			
Impact of SPI on practitioners at ward level	Ethnographic observations, interviews, and focus groups in acute medical wards	SPI1 hospitals	NA
Quality of care: acute medical care			
Quality of care of patients aged >65 with acute respiratory disease	Case note reviews (both explicit and holistic)	Control and SPI1 hospitals	Patient
Outcomes			
Adverse events in patients aged >65 with acute respiratory disease	Holistic case note review	Control and SPI1 hospitals	Patient
Hospital mortality in patients aged >65 with acute respiratory disease	Case note review	Control and SPI1 hospitals	Patient
Patient satisfaction	Questionnaire as used in NHS patient surveys	Control and SPI1 hospitals	Hospital

Source: Benning et al. (2011).

The evaluation report's findings say that senior staff were knowledgeable and enthusiastic about SPI. There was a small but significant effect in favour of the SPI hospitals in one of 11 dimensions of the staff questionnaire (organizational climate). Qualitative evidence showed only modest penetration of the SPI at the medical ward level. Recording of respiratory rate increased and use of a formal scoring system for patients with pneumonia increased. Of the five components to identify patients at risk of deterioration, there was little difference between the control and the SPI hospitals. There were no improvements in the proportion of prescription errors and no effects that could be attributed to SPI1 in generic areas (such as enhanced safety culture).

On some measures, the lack of effect could be because compliance was already high at the baseline (such as use of steroids in over 85 per cent of cases where indicated), but even when there was more room for improvement (such as in quality of medical history-taking), there was no significant additional net effect of SPI.

There were no changes over time or between control and SPI hospitals in errors or rates of adverse events in patients in medical wards. Mortality increased from 11 per cent (27) to 16 per cent (39) among controls and decreased from 17 per cent (63) to 13 per cent (49) among SPI1 hospitals, but the risk-adjusted difference was not significant. Poor care was a contributory factor in four of the 178 deaths identified by review of case notes. The survey of patients showed no significant differences apart from an increase in perception of cleanliness in the SPI hospitals.

Certainty about and generalizability of the outcomes

The research used a pre-defined protocol, quantified safety practices and independent case note reviewers who made observations across multiple hospitals. This reduced the risk of bias in comparisons. Observations across the different levels within the hospitals made possible 'triangulation' of qualitative and quantitative data and thus increased the certainty about the findings.

The comparisons with control hospitals increased the certainty that the outcomes were due to the intervention and not to other changes. Reproducing the principles and methods of the intervention would be possible, as many details are presented in other documents. But whether the results would be similar is unlikely as the context would be different with different quality payment and other changes.

Summary: strengths and weaknesses of the design in this example

This design involved comparisons with 'control' hospitals, and used a before/after 'difference in difference' approach to quantitative measurements. Most other large-scale evaluations rely on the hospitals' own quality project's data collection, but this study made more rigorous independent research assessments. One weakness, apart from the cost of the study, was that randomization was not used: the 'control' SPI1 hospitals might have had less scope for improvement, and controls might have had higher than average performance, particularly as half were also selected as future SPI phase 2 intervention sites. These four initial SPI hospitals were selected, not chosen at random. Agreement to participate in the evaluation could have had a motivating effect in SPI hospitals compared to control hospitals.

Example 9 Case evaluation of a programme for electronic summaries of patients' medical records (mixed methods)

This example evaluation used a different approach to evaluate a different and even larger-scale intervention to all UK NHS services: a national programme with activities which aimed to develop and implement centrally-stored electronic summaries of patients' medical records (Greenhalgh et al. 2010b). What was referred to in this evaluation as a summary care record (SCR) was a structured summary of patient data, held on a national database, and accessible to authorized staff over a secure internet connection. The SCR was not an electronic medical record (EMR), but was intended as a shared record of limited data about each patient – a good summary of the UK SCR is given by Wikipedia. A system called 'Health Space' was to have provided patients with access to their own SCR. The evaluation was of a programme to enable providers to input patient data to the SCR and to use it.

The evaluation aimed to answer three questions:

1 What is the usability, use, functionality, and impact of the summary care record (SCR), and what explains variation in its adoption and use?
2 How was the SCR programme shaped by influences at the macro, meso and micro levels?
3 What are the lessons for practice and policy?

The intervention evaluated

A major part of this evaluation was simply to describe the actions and arrangements at different organizational levels of the NHS which were made to establish the SCR and how they changed over time. There was a plan, but what was actually done to enable uptake of the SCR was significantly different.

The intervention was in a few areas at first and included information to patients about the programme and that they had the right to opt out of allowing their data to be uploaded. There was also information to providers, and assistance about details of what to upload, when and how. This intervention to the SCR was part of a wider programme to implement an electronic medical record in the public National Health Service (NHS) in England.

The evaluation design was a case evaluation, using mixed methods. It was informed by a 'utilization-focused evaluation', and a method for interpretive field studies in large-scale information systems (described in detail in Greenhalgh and Russell 2010). The former approach views complex programmes as having multiple stakeholders, each with different expectations of the programme and the evaluation (Patton 1997), and the latter approach is to make continuous, iterative comparison of findings in one part of the project with an emerging description of the whole programme (Klein and Myers 1999).

The design aimed to describe the intervention at a macro level (e.g. national policy, wider social norms and expectations), at a meso level (e.g. organizational processes and routines) and at a micro level (e.g. particular experiences of patients and professionals) using qualitative and quantitative data.

Outcomes measured and discovered

The findings reported included narrative descriptions of 'What stakeholders expected of the summary care record' and 'Implementing the programme' – the different actions and experiences of participants. Data reported about the use of summary care records were quantitative data: those collected and reported included:

proportion of patients with a summary care record; access rates to this record by providers (low); trends in accesses; and impact on consultation times.

Qualitative data included interviews with clinicians (which were used to explain the above). Ethnographic data on 214 clinical consultations showed that non-access of the SCR was for many different reasons, and shows some of the benefits of using it.

As regards certainty about and generalizability of the outcomes, the mixed methods and theory-informed design made it possible to explain the low use and identify improvements needed. The understanding of the programme was enhanced by applying socio-technical network theory to the data to understand it as a complex, dynamic and unstable socio-technical network. Using the data with this theory showed multiple interacting sub-networks, with individuals and organizations representing four different institutional 'worlds': political, clinical, technical and commercial.

Strengths and weaknesses of the design in this example

First, it needs to be noted that, separate from this evaluation, this implementation was widely viewed as limited, at best. Frankly, it was viewed by many, including this author as a sometimes UK patient and observer of the UK health scene, as a disaster. More objectively, this evaluation gave information about the implementation which was invaluable, independent and embarrassing for some, and which is highly relevant to any large-scale health information programme.

As regards the evaluation study design and its application, the literature review allowed pre-study identification of issues to explore and build a theoretical model to then inform data collection. The researchers propose:

> This enabled us to combine qualitative and quantitative techniques to highlight the competing conceptualizations and complex interdependencies of the SCR programme and to bring into frame numerous social, technical, ethical, and political explanations for why particular goals and milestones set by policy makers and implementation teams were or were not reached.

A possible weakness is that some users of this evaluation may not see the evidence as credible because the design was not a traditional one. The researchers suggest that some healthcare information systems researchers define rigour in terms of experimental or quasi-experimental studies of the 'deployment' of a technology and its 'impact' on predefined outcomes. They comment that:

> The profound epistemological differences and lack of dialogue between healthcare information systems research (led largely by doctors with an interest in information technology) and mainstream information systems research (led by interdisciplinary teams of organizational sociologists, computer scientists, and political scientists) have been highlighted previously.

Part III of this book gives a more detailed discussion of this design and the issues in evaluating digital health technologies and their implementation.

Evaluations of service performance

In the following, services are the intervention. We consider the performance of the service as an intervention, usually to patients, and ways to evaluate service performance. Perform means to carry out or accomplish something and performance is the manner in which something functions. For a service which you know, would you agree with the following definition of health service performance? 'Performance is the amount made or produced or done in relation to the resources used to make or produce or do it. It is output per unit of input' (Harper 1986).

To my mind, this is a definition of efficiency. It captures one aspect of performance but does not include effectiveness, quality and other aspects of performance which many people would want to include. One set of criteria which gives a basis for service evaluation is the 'famous five' performance criteria:

1 Economy: fewest resources or lowest cost (inputs).
2 Productivity: amount produced (output).
3 Efficiency: amount produced for the input (input/output).
4 Effectiveness: how well the service achieves the desired results (the change effected in the target, objectives met or needs/outcomes).
5 Quality: the degree to which the service satisfies patients, meets professionally assessed requirements and uses the fewest resources within regulations (requirements met).

The point here is not to put forward my definition of performance, but rather to show that evaluating performance means recognizing different perceptions of performance and being conscious of the criteria of performance which we are using.

As with any other intervention, value depends on whose perspective you take and the value criteria which are important to them. The evaluation methods to be used depend on the purpose of the evaluation. In this case, service performance evaluations are often to give information to buyers in order to help them choose a service: insurance companies, governments, employers or patients. The aim may be to help choose best value or check safety. Performance evaluations can be for managers of the service, for example, to help them improve or assess the impact of a recent change on performance and to make corrections to service strategy or organization.

Audit performance evaluations (APE)

A common performance evaluation method is to compare the service with a statement of what is expected of the service. This is the audit design described in Chapter 4. Accreditation or certification evaluations use this design. These evaluations collect data about the service which are relevant to assessing whether or how well the service is meeting standards or guidelines which are specified in the accreditation or certification manual.

One example is the accreditation system used by the Joint Commission for accreditation of healthcare organizations in the USA (JC 2013). The core of the system is the standards against which healthcare organizations are assessed, most of which state different processes or procedures which the organization is expected to have in place, and which are thought to contribute to quality outcomes. For example, one of the standards for evaluating academic medical centers (AMC) is: 'The organization understands and provides the required frequency and intensity of medical supervision for each type and level of medical student and resident trainee.' As regards the method for gathering data to assess whether the AMC meets this standard, the first is a self-assessment led by the quality officer at the AMC and then second is a site visit by a trained Joint Commission survey team, who are the external evaluators in this case. These evaluators use different methods to collect data to assess if the standards are met – the Joint Commission has experimented with remote surveys using a video camera carried by a local person to relay observations to help provide data for the assessment. Another performance audit assessment system, the European Foundation for Quality Management (EFQM) (1999), also uses standards or expectations and suggests methods for gathering data to evaluate the extent to which the expectations are met.

Single-service time-trend performance evaluation

These designs track the performance of a service over time – the comparison is, for example, performance every three months on different performance criteria.

The 'balanced scorecard' reporting system is a popular approach used to report a few carefully chosen dimensions of the service at regular intervals to management (Inamdar et al. 2002). The dimensions are chosen to enable management to pursue the objectives of the service and to balance sometimes conflicting demands. Typically they include indicators of financial performance, customer performance, internal processes, and internal development, or, for a clinical service functional outcomes, clinical outcomes, patient satisfaction and cost and utilization. This method in international health has been described by Peters et al. (2007), and a good guide to developing one for a healthcare service is given by NIII (2014).

There are two evaluation design challenges. First, to ensure the dimensions reported do give a balanced picture, and do not over-emphasize one aspect of performance in a way which might lead to actions which reduce the service's ability to meet its objectives over time. Second, to ensure that the data collected to inform performance on each dimension are valid data or measures of the dimension and give a comprehensive picture. This is often done by combining data from measures into one index number which summarizes performance on the one dimension.

Service-comparison performance evaluations

These compare the performance of a set of services at one time, in relation to one or more dimensions of service performance. There are many performance evaluation systems for comparing the performance of different types of health service. Examples are the systems by the US Medicare Program called Hospital Compare (2014), and TCWF (2014), and for the UK NHS the programmes are NHS (2014) and Dr Foster (2014). More guidance on performance evaluations of healthcare services can be found in Ozcan (2013). How valid these evaluation systems are for their purpose is discussed in Davis et al. (2013) and Ash et al. (2012). But the last word here goes to Florence Nightingale, commenting about mortality rates as a measure of hospital performance in 1863:

> If the function of a hospital were to kill the sick, statistical comparisons of this nature would be admissible. As, however, their proper function is to restore the sick to health as speedily as possible, the elements which really give information as to whether this is done or not, are those which show the proportion of sick restored to health, and the average time which has been required for this object.

Checklist for a performance evaluation

Here are some key questions to ask with regard to performance evaluation:

1 *Does it help* the people for whom the evaluation is designed do their work better? Which critical actions and decisions could be better informed by the performance evaluation?
2 *Control*: does the evaluation provide information about something which the users can do something about? Don't evaluate what users cannot do anything about.
3 *Process*: does the evaluation assess the process (which can be described and improved) or only outcomes? Information about outcome performance alone may not indicate actions to be taken.
4 *Three highs*: high volume, high cost and/or high risk. Concentrate attention on evaluating performance of services for these patient groups.
5 *Are the data quick and easy* to *gather and use* (ideally, have they already been collected)?
6 *Credible*: is it sufficiently reliable, valid, and sensitive for the purpose and user?
7 *Timely*: you want the least delay between event and presentation of evaluation (the 'Polaroid principle').
8 *Politically acceptable*: collection and use of the evaluation will not change the power balance between people in an unacceptable way (information is power).

Judge your existing or proposed performance evaluation against these criteria.

Excellent guides for selecting indicators for healthcare performance measurement are provided by Penchon (2014), and Damberg et al. (2011).

Conclusion

Interventions to health services as work organization need to be evaluated as interventions to subjects which are not only a collection of individuals – a hospital is more than the sum of the individuals working there. The subject in which the intervention aims to enable change is a social entity with explicit procedures and systems, and implicit norms and customs which affect what people do and will affect any intervention. These outlast individuals but are passed on by individuals' actions. Some multiple component interventions to services aim to change these features of these social entities. Some do not.

This chapter considered how this feature of the subjects of the intervention might affect the design of an intervention and of an evaluation of the intervention. It showed how certain evaluation designs given in Chapter 4 were modified to assess different interventions to health services: an intervention to intensive care units, then a large-scale safety programme to hospitals, then an intervention to health services to enable them to make and use electronic summaries of electronic medical records.

It also considered evaluation systems to assess the performance of health services and the three designs commonly used to assess performance: the audit design, the time-trend performance of a single service, and comparative performance of similar services.

8 Evaluating interventions to health systems and performance

Introduction

What is the difference between a health system and a health service? Both give health services to a population. It is true that most healthcare services can be considered as a set of services, such as those in a hospital or primary care centre. But these 'separate services' are not so separate – they are part of one organization: part of one hospital or one primary care centre. Examples of health systems are a nation's public healthcare and health service (e.g. in the UK, Spain and Italy), or an integrated service delivery system such as Kaiser Permanente in the USA, a Swedish county health system or the Veterans' Health Administration regional and national system.

Is a health system one organization in the same sense as a hospital or primary care centre is one organization? Might the differences be significant for how we intervene to change a health system as opposed to a health service? And might we need to use different or modified evaluation designs for evaluation interventions to health systems from those we use to evaluate interventions to health services? And are these differences because of the scope or scale of a health system compared to that of a health service?

Health systems are similar to most health services in that they are also a set of interconnected healthcare services. But they are not only larger – they often include a wider range of different services. This sometimes includes departments of public health and also a funding organization such as an insurance plan or public purchasing organization.

Perhaps more importantly for interventions and their evaluation is the connection between the organizations in a health system compared to the connections between services in a hospital or primary care centre. In health systems, the interconnection can be strong, where a set of primary – the hospital – and other services are designed to work together to provide healthcare and health promotion for a population (and Integrated Service Delivery System (ISDS)). Or it can be weak, where a set of public and private providers compete to provide services to a defined geographic population, such as the health system in one Australian state – here 'health system' means something different from what it means with a more integrated set of service: it is all the services in a geographic area or for a defined population.

This chapter considers designs to evaluate interventions to health systems, such as a change to the way hospitals and primary care services are paid. If the change was only to how only hospitals were paid, then this would be an intervention to a service which was considered in Chapter 7. It is the system-wide intervention that characterizes the interventions evaluated in this chapter.

The chapter also considers performance evaluations of health systems: there is no intervention, but the performance of a health system is evaluated. Usually the evaluation design of a system to compare performance uses different dimensions to assess the system's performance previously, or to other comparable systems, as, for example, with a hospital comparison website.

The chapter considers example evaluations of interventions to health systems which use evaluation designs which were described in Chapter 4. First, an example which uses realist evaluation design (Example 10), and this is followed by a discussion of approaches to evaluating health reforms as interventions to health systems. The designs for performance evaluation of a health system are considered which use single-case time trend performance evaluation and comparative performance evaluation.

Example 10 Formative realist case evaluation

This was an evaluation of a difficult-to-describe large-scale 'transformation' of health services in London (Greenhalgh et al. 2009) and the related report (Greenhalgh et al. 2008). The overall questions addressed were those considered in all realist evaluations, 'what works, for whom, under what circumstances?' and 'what are transferable lessons about effective change?' This second question arose because the users wanted information which showed how the changes applied were influenced by and in turn influenced the environment surrounding the 'transformation' intervention – the environment being such things as finance, resources, changes in policy and related services.

The intervention evaluated was a change programme to a public healthcare system to make stroke, kidney, and sexual health services more 'efficient, effective, and patient-centred'. Therefore, it was not an evaluation of comprehensive healthcare reform, which would have involved many other interventions in the 'transformation' activities.

The design was a formative realist case evaluation, which was informed by the realist context–intervention–mechanism theory (one type of programme theory). It used mixed data sources and collection methods of ethnographic observation, semi-structured interviews, and document analysis. These were applied in the evaluation in a 'pragmatic and reflexive manner to build a picture of the case and follow its fortunes over the three-year study period'.

The design uses inductive interpretation of the data to build a theory: it started with the broad model of context–intervention–mechanism/outcomes and developed this model using data bit by bit from the different data collection methods. It used methods to increase validity such as noting participants' reactions to interpretations, triangulating data sources, and seeking disconfirmations for initial interpretations. The aim was to identify which mechanisms are triggered in certain contexts by the intervention, to then result in service changes, which were thought to improve patient outcomes (i.e. an influence pathway or causal chain in the programme theory). The steps taken to do this were:

- Organizing primary data and producing initial thematic summaries of these, and repeating this at a later time to document changes.
- Presenting, criticizing and adopting particular interpretations of actions and events within the research team and also with stakeholders.
- Testing interpretations by seeking disconfirming or contradictory data.
- Considering other interpretations of the same findings.
- Using cross-case comparisons to consider how the same mechanism such as 'integrating services across providers' was carried out in different contexts and produced different outcomes, which then made it possible to infer the 'generative causality' of these different contexts.

Findings

The findings were reported in relation to six 'mechanisms of change' and associated 'lessons' for others seeking similar changes. For example, Mechanism 1 was described as:

> Integrating Services across Providers: through establishing boundary-spanning roles, shared guidelines, protocols, pathways, IT systems and common data sets, developing networks and supporting networking.

As regards 'lessons', these were reported as follows: that efforts to achieve integration across providers are more likely to succeed when:

- Relationships between organizations are trusting, with a history of collaboration, and compatible values rather than competition.
- Approaches to integration are imaginative, locally responsive, negotiable, and supported by technology rather than rigid and driven by technology.
- External incentives are designed to reward collaborative performance and do not make organizations compete.
- The strategy for integration includes both 'soft' and 'hard' approaches.
- Solutions are participatory rather than developed by one party and imposed on others.

The following represents the context–mechanism–outcome understanding presented by the study for the first of the six mechanisms (the context is 'enabling and constraining factors that appeared to make each mechanism more or less likely to produce a desired outcome in any particular set of circumstances') (Figure 8.1).

The other mechanisms of change also had associated 'lessons', but only three were presented in the study 'for length of article reasons'. The others were: Mechanism 2: Finding and using evidence; Mechanism 3: Involving service users in the modernization effort; Mechanism 4: Supporting self-care; Mechanism 5: Developing the workforce; and Mechanism 6: Extending the range of services.

Outcomes are described in more detail in another report and include 'hard' (evidence-based protocols; extended opening hours; shorter waiting lists;

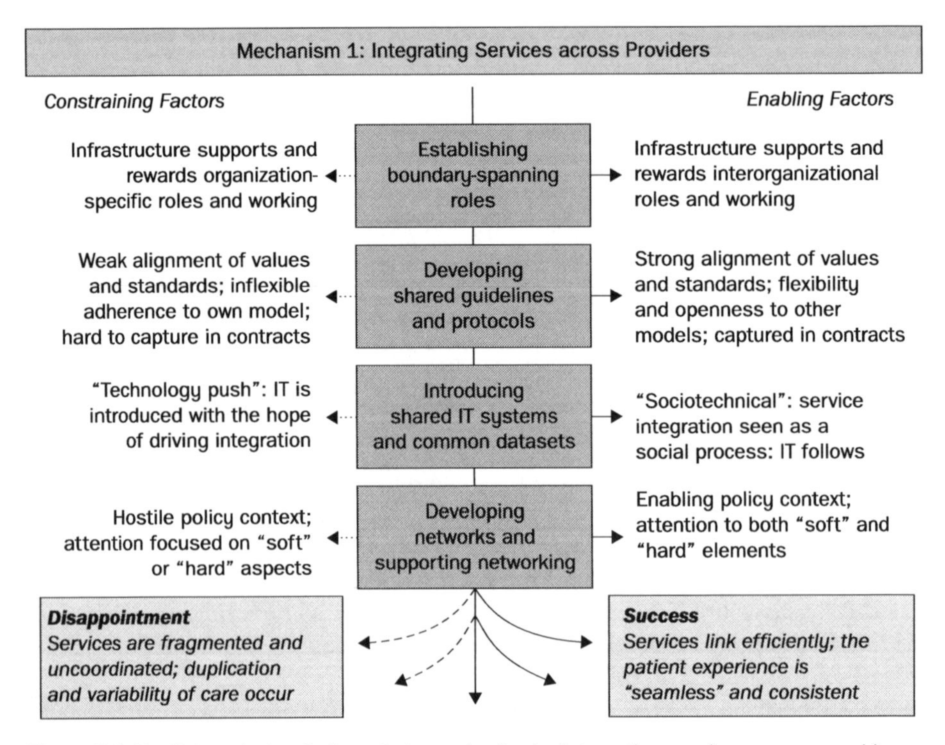

Figure 8.1 Realist analysis of attempts to modernize by integrating services across providers
Source: Greenhalgh et al. (2009).

governance structures for inter-organizational working) and 'soft' (improved staff attitudes and motivation, greater user satisfaction, and what one senior manager described as a 'precious, extraordinary' cultural shift) (Greenhalgh et al. 2008).

Certainty about, and generalizability of the findings

The purpose of the evaluation was to inform others about effective strategies for similar changes, as well as to feed back learning to the implementers.

Methods often used within the qualitative and mixed method researcher communities were applied to maximize certainty about the outcomes. If we trust that the researchers appropriately applied these accepted methods, then certainty about these findings would have been increased: interpretive case study methods, with a team culture which challenged each other to apply these methods. This is done by carefully defining and justifying the 'case', 'immersion in the case' (i.e. spending enough time at the field site to understand what is happening), systematic data collection and analysis, reflexivity in both researchers and research participants, developing theory iteratively as emerging data are analysed, seeking disconfirming cases and alternative explanations and defending interpretations to both the research participants and academic peers.

The generalizability is increased by providing details of the change actions and of the context. This allows others to assess whether, if they applied these actions in their setting, they would be likely to get similar results. The description of the 'mechanisms' or change principles, and how they were triggered by the intervention in the setting enables others to try to reproduce the mechanism in their different setting using possibly different interventions.

The discussion section of the study elaborates on the design, and proposes 'a greater understanding of these underlying mechanisms will help inform similar change programs in the future' and that the researchers:

> deliberately not passed judgment on the program's overall 'success' . . . If a team sets out to achieve X but along the way learns things or encounters challenges that convince it that Y is a more appropriate (or practicable) goal, then it will have 'succeeded' if it achieves something approaching Y.

The researchers comment that:

> Building the evaluation criteria for expensive, large-scale change programs on such shifting sands is relatively controversial when judged by conventional clinical research criteria, which define 'rigor' as the systematic pursuit of well-defined goals, objective measurement of progress, and robust accountability procedures.

Strengths and weaknesses of the design in this example

The design gives a narrative understanding of the process of change in an environment, rather than showing a few measured outcomes attributed to a change as is more usual in evaluations. It can answer some questions about implementation and necessary conditions, but does not give clear-cut answers to the 'did patients benefit?' question. This is because other changes are not controlled for and the research resources and data focus were on process, not later end outcomes. The design is also dependent on the researcher's experience and skills with the interpretive methods, and the rigour with which the research team apply the methods. This true for all designs, but perhaps more so with this type of design.

The discussion section in the paper comments on the methods, as it is one of the first studies to use a design of this type. The researchers report that identifying the mechanisms of change was far more difficult than the text-book on realist evaluation suggests (Pawson and Tilley 1997). They concluded that researchers 'must anticipate the mismatch between the realist evaluation's assumption that a set of more or less well-defined "mechanisms of change" can be articulated and tested and the empirical reality in which these mechanisms may prove stubbornly hard to nail'. Alternative 'mechanisms of change' explanations could be proposed and it was not possible in this study to decide which was operating. This does raise questions about whether other evaluators would have produced similar findings using the same methods and about the certainty of the attribution of the findings to the transformation changes, rather than to something else.

Other researchers have used this design and found that 'surfacing theories of change', did not enable an understanding of the power dynamics among different groups. They recommended the design also draws on other theories to document and understand the politics of change (e.g. neo-institutional theory (Barnes et al. 2003)). A further comment is made about the participatory or action-role of the researcher-evaluators (Guba and Lincoln 1989; Patton 1997; Øvretveit 2002).

This study was also action research in that the researchers fed back to the implementers the interim findings. They also discussed and tested the ideas about mechanisms and context with different actors, which also was likely to change the programme. The researchers argue that the design is thus incompatible with a detached objectivist approach to research.

Moore (2012) gives a summary of the limitations of and issues with the approach:

1 Distinguishing between context and mechanism.
2 Is there an end point?
3 When to 'close'?
4 Time-consuming.
5 Can realist evaluation studies be replicated?
6 How does realist evaluation differ from traditional mediator/moderator analysis?

Evaluating health reforms to health systems

The above was an example of an evaluation design applied to the evaluation of a discrete set of interventions to a complex regional health system. Some might call the transformation evaluated a 'reform', because this term has a wide meaning applied to many types of change to large-scale health and healthcare systems. More often, a health or healthcare reform is a more comprehensive and longer-term set of change interventions to a range of services.

One health reform is the changes introduced by the US Patient Protection and Affordable Care Act of 2010 (PPACA 2010). This makes health insurance available to more Americans, and in one respect is a limited type of reform to healthcare financing. In fact, the ACA 2010 covers many types of change to finance, healthcare and health promotion, including many quality improvement interventions, to be introduced in stages over eight years. How much is implemented is a question of debate, but how would we evaluate such an 'intervention'? Would we break it down into different parts and evaluate each separately and aggregate these evaluations in one final evaluation report? Would this capture the synergy between the parts or lose synergy if the parts are not implemented?

This section of the chapter does not give a definitive answer. And that is not only because space is short. Rather, it provides some discussion of methods for evaluating a health reform and where to go for more guidance and resources on this subject.

Why evaluate a reform?

The reasons to evaluate a reform before it starts are to assess whether it is feasible, to predict problems and to help plan how to implement it. This is 'formative evaluation' and can be done by piloting the change in one area, or by making a 'paper evaluation', which draws on evidence from evaluations of similar changes elsewhere.

During a reform, the reasons to make an evaluation are to help make corrections during the implementation. After the reform, an evaluation helps to explain the lessons for future changes or reforms, and contributes to scientific knowledge which could help the reformers explain, understand or predict the effects of large-scale changes. A more immediate reason is to hold politicians and managers to account for the changes which they made, or did not make.

Evaluating a reform follows the steps described in Chapter 3 and usually involves:

- describing the reform 'instrument' (e.g. a law, which states intentions) and the implementation process (i.e. what was actually done);
- gathering data about changes in health service performance and possibly also in health (outcome data);
- assessing whether these data really are outcomes of the reform (i.e. assessing the extent to which the reform caused or influenced the changes registered in the outcome indicators).

The aim is often to do the following:

- present evidence of the results of the reform;
- describe the process of implementing the reform;
- assess the strengths and weaknesses of the reform as implemented and judge the value of the results (in relation to the criteria of valuation used in the evaluation);
- recommend improvements.

Examples of reforms

The mental health decentralization reforms in Norway and Sweden in the early 1990s were initiated by laws changing the responsibilities of counties and smaller communes within the counties. A law transferred responsibilities for general care for people with mental health problems from the counties 'downwards' to communes. Like other reforms, it was an 'intervention' which was planned and had a managed implementation process, though there were different views about how well this was done.

In most reforms, the intention is to change the organization, the procedures, financing methods and other 'things'. These are termed the 'immediate subject' or 'target' of the reform intervention – the thing which the intervention acts on directly and aims to change in the short term. But there is often an aim beyond changing health organizations or financing methods – the long-term aim is often to make services better for patients (e.g. more accessible and responsive) or to improve patients' health or well-being. Following the concepts described in Chapter 2, these are the intended 'ultimate beneficiaries' of the change.

Not all healthcare reforms have this aim. For those that do, the intervention does not work directly on the ultimate beneficiaries (patients or the population) but works through changing the immediate subject (health organization) in order to achieve the ultimate benefits of better health. The objectives are usually to save money, improve quality, increase production, efficiency or effectiveness. There are often multiple purposes, such as to reduce public expenditure, increase efficiency and choice, and make services more responsive to patients.

The complexity of health reforms is a challenge to the evaluators, as they need to describe exactly what the reform is which is implemented, not what the reform was on paper. The following gives an example of the difficulty of defining a reform:

> We are introducing a change to our procedures, which is intended to change how our personnel act, in order to change how patients take care of themselves. The aim is to improve the health of the population. We do not expect other significant changes to occur, but some may be unavoidable.

Which of the changes is the intervention which we evaluate? All of them? Which other changes might the evaluators study? The statement has the advantage of describing different components and some components may be viewed as part of the reform to be evaluated. It can be used to map a reform sequence or causal chain model – these are the methods that evaluators use to define a reform.

Choice of design

A key step is choosing a design that is most likely to answer the user's questions, given the resources and other constraints on the evaluation. There are four designs which have been used to evaluate health reforms. The most common is a before/after single case design.

1 Implementation designs

These designs do not look at the effects of the reform but describe what was done in implementing the reform. The evaluators decide which aspects of the implementation to examine and use interviews and documentation to follow or reconstruct the process. They report on strengths and weaknesses of the process, and make explicit the criteria used to assess the process. For example, one criterion might be whether all stakeholder groups were involved. The evaluator may use descriptive case study methods (Yin 1989) and also draw on an ideal and an actual model of the implementation process to help construct their description.

2 Comparing achievements with reform objectives

This design compares the intended goals of the reform with the extent to which these are achieved. Using this design to evaluate a decentralized mental health reform would mean finding out the intended goals from documents. Then deciding which data would make it possible to judge the extent to which these goals were met, and collecting and presenting these data. In effect, it means thinking of the goals as the only criterion for valuation of the reform. This may or may not include looking at the ultimate effects of the reform on people with mental health problems or who are at risk: it would depend on whether this was a stated goal.

Some reform intentions do not mention improving health as a goal. If so, this design would not be suitable for some users who had this as a value criterion. The evaluator may also feel that there were missing goals and value criteria which should be used in evaluating the reform, such as the effect on equity of access.

One of the challenges of using this type of design is that goals are often general principles or aspirations and it is not clear which data would give evidence of the extent to which the goals were met. Evaluators usually have to translate goals into what can be measured. Users or other stakeholders may not accept that the measures are valid indicators of goal achievement, so it is wise to discuss these with the users of the evaluation at the planning stage. Note that doing this may help users more clearly to define the objectives, which itself changes the reform.

3 Before/after design

This design describes the reform implementation process but also gathers data before, and then after the reform has been proceeding for enough time to have an effect. Which data to collect before and after, and the length of time would depend on the value criteria against which the reform is to be assessed: common criteria are costs, efficiency, access, equity, quality and service comprehensiveness.

The data to be collected would also depend on the evaluation timescale: if the evaluation results are required soon after the start of the reform (e.g. one or two years), then only some effects might be expected, for example, effects on health providers and the organization.

Is this design not possible when there are no 'before' data available, for example, on costs? Not necessarily, because the evaluator could interview different stakeholders and collect their views about any before/after differences. The aim is to reach plausible explanations or conclusions rather than statistical probabilistic proof of causality.

4 Comparing one site with one or more others implementing the reform

This comparative design gathers data about different sites or areas implementing the same reform. It can be used cross-nationally to compare similar types of reform, for example, purchaser–provider reforms or market reforms, or within one country to compare different areas. What is compared? This depends on the evaluation users' interests and value criteria. It usually involves comparing the implementation process at different places and using the comparison to try to discover factors which helped or hindered the speed and depth of the implementation.

In deciding on a design, consider whether there is the possibility of piloting the reform changes in one area or organization. This may allow a comparative study. Another possibility is that there may be areas or organizations which have not implemented the reform, or where penetration of the change has been low or slow, and which could serve as a comparison site or a control site, or which could allow a 'natural experiment'. Table 8.1 shows a model of a healthcare reform for identifying the data required for an evaluation.

Questions for deciding which design and data-gathering methods to use

- Who is the evaluation for?
- Which decisions or actions could the evaluation inform or make a difference to?
- Which data are readily available and reliable?

The last item above refers to data about what was done, about before and after effects on providers, patients or populations. (Sources are documents, statistics, and people. Which experts can advise on or give you the data and help you assess and interpret these data?)

Practical advice for evaluating a healthcare reform

- Focus on specific aspects of the reform and map the 'reform causal-change-chain'.
- For a complex multiple component reform, make separate evaluations of each component of the reform, and later assess whether there is a mutual reinforcing effect between the components.
- Use the stated aims of reform and your ideas about likely effects to generate hypotheses to test: this helps to focus on which data/indicators to gather.
- The ideal is the enemy of the good and the feasible: realistically assess, in relation to the time and personnel you have, which data you must collect and what is easily available.
- Find and ask experts to get or advise you on where the data are and their validity and reliability.
- List which interviewees are accessible (allowing for appointment cancellations and the need to follow new trails as you go).
- Use formal contacts to introduce the evaluation and yourself, and to get interviewee and expert cooperation (the time saving outweighs the danger of bias and concealment, especially if you 'triangulate' the data from different sources).
- List factors other than the reform which are affecting the subject, patients and populations, and think about how to judge the different effects of the reform (plan the design).

Table 8.1 Model of a healthcare reform for identifying the data required for an evaluation

The intervention				**Outcomes (intended and unintended)**	
Environment of reform and pressures	Reform aims, instrument, and content	>>> Reform implementation process>>>	Target of reform instrument	Effect on target (short-term outcome)	Impact on patients, on populations (long-term outcome)

How good is this evaluation of a health reform?

Table 8.2 shows a list of questions to assess an evaluation of a health reform or intentional change

Table 8.2 Questions to assess an evaluation of a health reform or intentional change

	Data (Score 0–5)	Design (Score 0–5)	Relevance (Score 0–5)
Description of the reform	How good was the description of the actual implementation of the change? (The criterion for a 'good' description is that someone else could repeat it, and that the sources are accurate, i.e. position and time documented) How good is the description of the intended changes? (E.g. from official documents) How good is the description of the context to the change? (To enable someone to judge (a) if a similar context is present for them, (b) whether factors other than the change might have caused any before/after differences which were reported)	How good are the methods used to gather data and to describe the intervention? What is the likelihood of an average professional using these methods being able to create a 'good' description of the implementation process?	How similar is the intervention to one which you are implementing or could implement? How similar is the context to your context?
Effects	Are there before/after data, which are valid, and reliable? Are the other data about possible effects reliable and valid?	Were data gathered about all important and possible effects?	Are these the effects which are of interest in your situation?
Explanation	How probable is it that the before/after differences are due to the intervention?	Internal validity Are all other explanations for the before/after differences considered (other than the intervention)? Have these explanations been satisfactorily excluded? (E.g. by planning controls before, or by retrospective assessment of their possible influence)	External validity How likely are similar effects in your situation if you applied this intervention in your context? (Is it valid to generalize these findings to your situation – what is different and are these differences significant?)

Evaluations of system performance

So far the chapter has considered evaluations of interventions to health systems. In this last section, we consider evaluations of health system where a specific intervention is not being evaluated. The aims of health system performance evaluations vary: some are to provide health system managers with data to help improve performance, some are to provide purchasers with assessments about how the health system is performing, and some are to provide patients or consumers with information which can be useful if they are free to choose between two or more health systems.

The three designs for performance evaluation are: (1) audit; (2) single-case time trend performance evaluation; and (3) comparative performance evaluation. For all performance evaluations, the three key questions are: who is the evaluation for? What do they need to know to act differently and better (their value criteria)? And, which data could provide this actionable knowledge?

Audit performance evaluations (APE)

This design compares the health system with a statement of what is expected of the system. For example, in the USA, an employer looking to provide healthcare benefits for employees might consider directly contracting a health system. That is, if there is an entity called a health system in the employer's area that provides the range of services which employees need. One thing the employer wants to know is whether the health system provides the services needed, so the employer might use an evaluator to write a specification of which services are needed and compare this specification to what the local health system provides.

Another example from the USA of this design is the NCQA accreditation of an ACO (NCQA 2013). An ACO is an accountable care organization, which is networks of doctors and hospitals that assume financial responsibility for managing the healthcare of a specific group of patients, for example, patients with chronic conditions in a particular area. If the ACO is able to provide lower overall healthcare costs of their patients while also improving the quality of their care, they will receive financial rewards. NCQA is the not-for-profit national council for quality assurance in the USA. They provide an accreditation of an ACO's ability to coordinate care and be accountable for the high-quality, efficient, patient-centred care that is expected from ACOs. Such an accreditation is an example of an audit evaluation of one limited type of health system – an ACO for a specific population.

Single-case time trend performance evaluation

These designs track the performance of a health system over time. An example of how such an evaluation of a regional US health system performance might be done would be to use routinely collected and reported Healthcare Effectiveness Data and Information Set (HEDIS) data about the health system and compare these at different times. The HEDIS data are used by US purchasers to measure performance on important dimensions of care and service. The data are 75 measures across eight domains of care (NCQA 2013). One example is the rate of patients who were hospitalized and discharged alive after an acute heart attack, who had received treatment with beta-blockers for six months after discharge. Whether the evaluator would use any of these data would depend on the evaluation user's needs.

Service-comparison performance evaluation

These designs compare the performance of a set of services at one time, in relation to one or more dimensions of service performance. There are many performance evaluation systems for comparing the performance of different types of health service. In the USA, the HEDIS data are widely reported by health systems and can be used for performance comparisons. Few systems report a comprehensive set of data. The most developed and longest-running systems report quality and safety data but not costs and so value assessment is not possible. One of the best systems is the US compare system, run by the Commonwealth Fund (TCWF 2014).

Finally, the Institute for Healthcare Improvement (IHI) 'triple aim initiative' provides a useful set of criteria and measures for evaluating a health system (Stiefel and Nolan 2012). A good overview of performance evaluation systems in public healthcare is given by Nuti et al. (2012), which also provides an evaluation of the effectiveness of the system developed in Tuscany, Italy.

Conclusion

Health systems include health services, but are organized subjects of a different order to a health service. An intervention to a nation's health system or a regional integrated healthcare system needs to be evaluated in a different way from an intervention to a hospital, primary care centre, or to a information service to patients. This chapter considered how one design and the principles outlined in Chapter 4 were modified to evaluate an intervention to a health system: a large-scale 'transformation' of health services in London. It also considered other designs possible for evaluating health reforms – the latter being an intervention to a health system which covers many comprehensive and limited large-scale changes. It concluded by considering performance evaluation of health systems and some of the approaches and examples of such systems.

9 Evaluating population health interventions and public health service performance

Introduction

Health education and health promotion – two types of population health intervention – have outcomes which take time to appear. The health of a community or population is influenced by many things other than these interventions. The time delay and the other influences can make evaluating these interventions more difficult than evaluating a surgical treatment or a rehabilitation service. The evaluation principles and methods already considered need to be adapted to evaluate these interventions. We often need to use a programme theory or causal chain to map how the intervention activities work through different stages to influence the health of the population. This chapter uses examples to show the variations in methods for evaluating population health interventions and some of the issues to consider.

Chapter 8 considered health systems. Surely a health system is a 'population health intervention'? Why, then, a separate chapter on 'evaluating population health interventions'? One answer is, because health education and health promotion programmes are often not provided by healthcare professionals, and they need different methods for their evaluation. It is true that some health systems also provide non-healthcare services to prevent illness and promote health. But these may be a small part of the set of these services. Health education and health promotion programmes intervene for communities or populations in a different way from the way that healthcare services intervene for patients.

Healthcare services do contribute to the health of a population, but the science of public health has found that other factors are often more important than health services. Methods to evaluate non-healthcare interventions to communities and populations are often different from those for evaluating health systems. This chapter considers these different methods, as well as how to evaluate routine public health services which are not healthcare services, such as disease monitoring and infection control services.

Hawe and Potvin (2009) define population interventions as policies or programmes that change the distribution of health risk by addressing the underlying social, economic and environmental conditions. They include programmes or policies designed and developed in the health sector, but which often include actions involving education, housing or employment. Many of the challenges and possible designs for evaluation are described in Waters et al. (2006), Potvin et al. (2001) and Hawe et al. (1990).

The chapter first gives an example evaluation. This is taken from a long-running and well-evaluated health promotion programme, starting in the early 1970s in Finland to prevent heart disease. It then gives a framework to help plan such evaluations. The chapter finishes by showing how to evaluate the performance of a routine public health service (not a public healthcare service) such as a department of public health in a region.

Example evaluation of an intervention to a community to prevent heart disease

North Karelia was formerly a rural farming community in Finland near the Russian border, where the inhabitants began to experience high rates of heart disease in the late 1960s. The question addressed by the Puska (Puska et al. 1985) evaluation was, does a community-based prevention programme reduce the risk factors for heart disease?

The intervention evaluated was a mass media campaign, and assistance to health and community groups to provide health education information to individuals and to make changes in the social and physical environment to motivate and maintain behavioural change.

The evaluation design was an experimental comparative case design, with the other case being a similar nearby community. Independent random samples of adults were surveyed before the intervention in 1972 and again five and ten years later. The surveys asked questions about health knowledge, attitudes, and behaviour, and included an examination to measure height, weight, blood pressure and cholesterol. Finally, mortality rates for the two communities were compared.

The data gathered were informed by a programme theory. This was that targeting individuals' knowledge and attitudes, and providing social and environmental support for behavioural change would lead individuals to reduce their risk factors for cardiovascular disease. The authors state that the theory of how the programme would work was only partially developed at the start because there were few theories related to community interventions. Thus, the evaluation tracked individuals' knowledge, attitudes, and behaviour – the most developed part of the programme theory – while documenting programme-related activities in the community through a process evaluation.

The findings

The findings were that knowledge of risk factors increased slightly in North Karelia. The evaluators report no major changes in health attitude measures, with little difference between the two communities. Over a ten-year period, a reduction in smoking and blood pressure was found in North Karelia. A reduction in serum cholesterol was found for men in North Karelia. Coronary heart disease (CHD) mortality also decreased by 22 per cent compared to 12 per cent in the comparison community. For CHD incidence and mortality rates, the maximal difference in favour of the intervention area was observed some five–eight years after its start (Puska et al. 1995). For cancer mortality, a net reduction in favour of North Karelia was observed later, five–ten years after the intervention started.

The lack of change in individuals' knowledge and attitudes led the authors to attribute the success of the project more to its community organization aspects than to the project's efforts to target individuals. They believe that health education messages disseminated through the media and opinion leaders gradually created an environment promoting healthier lifestyles and that these environmental changes then gradually influenced individual behaviour.

One strength of the evaluation was the timescale – this was necessary in order to register the effects of the sustained intervention on the intermediate and ultimate outcomes measured. Another was the causal-chain programme theory which hypothesized how the intervention would influence the intermediate outcomes of knowledge and attitudes. Discovering little change in these, but also observing the overall impact of the programme on health outcomes, gave support to changing the focus to the social and cultural environments in which individuals live, rather than to changing only individual knowledge and attitudes.

Table 9.1 summarizes the staged outcome data collected in the causal chain of the programme theory which hypothesized how the community-based intervention could work through different influences to reduce heart disease.

Frameworks to help evaluation of interventions to population health

Concepts and frameworks which help evaluations of interventions to population health derive from a critique of the limitations of the research evaluation model from

Table 9.1 Simple programme theory of the North Karelia community-based intervention

Evaluation design	Programme theory	Stage outcome data	Findings
Programme community compared to nearby comparison community Independent random samples of adults preintervention (T1), 5 years post-intervention (T2), and 10 years post-intervention (T3)	Change in individuals' knowledge and attitudes and providing social and environmental support for behaviour change . . . may influence >>> reductions in individuals' risk factors (smoking, serum cholesterol, and blood pressure) . . . may influence >>> reduced mortality at population level	Self-reports of knowledge, attitudes and behaviour Physical examination measuring height, weight, blood pressure, and cholesterol mortality	Knowledge of risk factors increased, but change was only slightly higher in programme community No major changes in health attitudes Net reduction in smoking for programme community (27%) Net reduction in serum cholesterol for programme in men Net reduction for blood pressure From 1974 to 1979, coronary heart disease mortality decreased (22% in programme vs. 12% in comparison community)

biomedicine (Øvretveit 2013). This proposes such models do not give sufficient recognition that population health interventions are:

- a series of actions carried out by human beings with varying intensity and quality (protocols often cannot be enforced);
- to influence other human beings (who have choice, and are exposed to competing influences);
- working in a changing social, economic and political situation.

The desired effects depend on the intervention actions being carried out, as well as the social conditions that support the actions: the degree to which the actions can be fully and consistently carried out depends on the conditions 'surrounding' the actors, for example, support, resources, time, knowledge, skills, etc.

The effects of these actions also depend on conditions that help or hinder the actions to have the desired results (e.g. media or cultural influences that contradict or complement the actions and which interact with the actions at different times).

The sustainability of health promotion interventions and their results depend more on the surrounding conditions than for many other interventions: short-term evaluations are less sensitive to the role of surrounding conditions and how they change. To understand which conditions are necessary for implementation and for the desired effects, it does not always help to 'control these out' as 'confounders'. It may be better to understand how they can have an influence.

These ideas can be summarized by describing many health promotion programmes as complex social interventions, carried out under changing conditions which both help and hinder the intervention and its effects. These surrounding conditions become more influential the longer the programme continues or after the recipients of the programme are no longer exposed to it.

Concepts

The following concepts help to describe health promotion and education programmes in ways that allow more effective planning and evaluation.

- *Intervention*: an action carried out to effect a change in a person, population or organization – the intervention influences them to think or behave differently than they would otherwise.
- *Interventionist actors*: the health promotion or department of public health personnel carrying out actions to inform, educate and influence the public, politicians, providers and others.
- *Mediating actors*: the people whom health promotion implementers inform, educate, or influence, so that these actors are better able to inform, educate, or influence others (e.g. the Department of Health Promotion teaches health personnel how to educate and work with young people regarding 'sensible drinking').
- *Ultimate recipients*: the people whose health and well-being are at risk.
- *Intervention actions*: these are of two types: *direct*: actions directed at the ultimate recipients (e.g. quit-smoking telephone line, media campaign) or *indirect*: actions

directed at mediating actors, with the intention that they influence the ultimate recipients (e.g. course on sexuality for teachers, on smoking prevention for GPs).

- *Conditions*: factors outside of the intervention that affect the capability of people to carry out the new actions, and which contribute to the effects (i.e. the helping or hindering conditions).

An evaluation framework to take account of the 'conditionality of results'

The evaluation model which follows states that evaluations need to do the following:

1. *Describe the programme*, how it was carried out and how it changed and compare this to the plan (correspondence, and degree of implementation).
2. *Describe the conditions* under which the programme was carried out and how these changed (using a theory of which conditions could be important in helping or hindering the 'implementation' of the programme and which could be necessary to create the desired effects).
3. *Collect data about results*: both people's perceptions of what difference the programme made and objective data.
4. *Explain the data results*: consider other explanations for the results, and assess the possible influence of the programme actions and conditions in accounting for the results.
5. *Make explicit the programme theory* held by the originators and participants about which actions and conditions are important (the environment–action–effect combination).
6. *Compare this theory* with the evidence from the evaluation to modify the programme theory.

Other guidance for evaluations

An alternative but similar framework to the above is described by Rootman et al. (1997). Fawcett et al. (1997), cited in Rootman and McQueen (1997), describe an approach to evaluating community initiatives for health and development as do Francisco et al. (1993).

The RE-AIM framework has proved useful for guiding evaluations of the implementation of health promoting and population health programmes (RE-AIM 2014) and for evaluating environmental change for population health (King et al. 2010). The framework proposes collecting data about each of the following:

- *Reach*: What was the participation rate among eligible individuals and the representativeness of the participants?
- *Effectiveness/efficacy*: What impact did the intervention have on primary outcomes of interest, quality of life and were there potential negative impacts?
- *Adoption*: What was the participation rate among settings and the representativeness of the setting participants?
- *Implementation*: Was the intervention delivered as intended? What were the time and costs of the intervention?

- *Maintenance*: What were the long-term effects of the programme on the outcomes six months or more after the intervention phase concluded? To what extent did the intervention become part of routine organizational practice and policy?

As regards evaluating the capacity of a community or programme to deliver effective health promotion, two useful tools are a checklist by Woodard et al. (2004), and indicators to help assess capacity building given by Hawe et al. (2000). Quality indicators for health promotion programmes are discussed in Ader et al. (2001). Simple guidance for assessing costs and benefits of health promotion is given in Haycox (1994).

Evaluating public health service performance

Chapter 8 considered how to evaluate the performance of a health system. It described some of the data about population health status which might be used to do so. These data and similar methods can also be used to evaluate the performance of a public health service, such as a department of public health. But other data are needed because the aims and impact of a public health service are different from those of a health system. Outcomes are longer-term and more difficult to attribute to the public health services rather than something else.

A public health service is a specific service, such as a health and disease monitoring and reporting service or a comprehensive set of public health services provided by one department or organization. A public health service may also include more than one specific service, but fall short of providing a comprehensive range of public health services, so the term covers specific services to comprehensive services and everything in between.

As always, the evaluation starts by defining the users' needs and employs this to decide the design and the data to be collected to meet those needs. The following considers different designs and data for different users' questions, which could include: what difference is this department of health making to the health of the population? How could I, as a manager of a public health service, improve our performance? How should we redistribute resources between different sub-services in our department of public health so as to use resources for the maximum health return?

The performance of a public health service could be considered in relation to different criteria and in relation to inputs, processes and outputs as shown in the NIPOO model in Chapter 2. As regards efficiency, costs and user satisfaction, similar criteria and methods to those used to evaluate healthcare services might be used. But different data would need to be collected about the processes of the service, its outputs and outcomes, and its quality.

Monitoring, measurement and evaluation of a public health service

To help think about how to evaluate a public health service, it is useful to re-visit the distinction in Chapter 1 between monitoring, measurement and evaluation. We can monitor a public health service by checking it is doing what is expected, for example, by using reports from the service. We can measure different aspects of the service by collecting quantitative data about the inputs to the service, its processes, and its outputs. But evaluation requires comparisons. Depending on the purpose, we may compare data over time or with similar services. It also may require us to identify and assess the outcomes of a public health service and this may call for a programme theory to map the influence pathways from the service activities to different short- and longer-term outcomes.

Data about community health

The general principle of 'do not collect data which you cannot attribute to the intervention' is especially important when considering performance evaluations of public health services. This is because changes in data about population health status will be influenced by many factors other than the public health services. So any data need to be linked via a theoretical pathway to the activities of the service. The positive side is that most departments of public health provide as one of their services data on the health status of the population. They are well placed both to consider whether or how health outcomes reflected in these data might be related to the department's activities, as well as having insight into the validity and reliability of the data.

Given this above qualification about attribution, there are a number of sources and databases in most countries which might provide data for evaluating the outcomes of a public health department – comparatively over time, or with similar services. Stiefel and Nolan (2012) provide a guide for measuring the triple aims of improving population health, improving the patient experience of care, and reducing per capita cost. Their discussion of population health measures can give a starting point for selecting measures for an evaluation of some public health services for two reasons: it is simple and clear, but also more health organizations are starting to use the triple aims as a strategic direction tool and measuring the public health service in relation to this shows the services' relevance to this overall strategy. This would be especially important if the public health service were part of a public health system which had adopted the triple aims as its strategy.

Two kinds of data are self-reports and more objective physiological, mortality or morbidity data. General population surveys that ask questions about health and function, such as those used in census data, might register the effects of some public health activities.

Designs for evaluating public health service performance

These data can be used in any of the three designs noted in Chapter 8 to evaluate the service and the system performance.

- *Audit design*: for example, the US Public Health Accreditation Board provides a set of standards for accrediting a department of public health, which could be used as a basis for a low-cost audit evaluation of the service (PHAB 2013).

- *Single-service time trend performance evaluation*: one design which is sometimes used is to track indicators of performance of one service or department at regular intervals. As described in earlier chapters, a 'balanced scorecard' for the service or department could be developed to guide the choice of a limited set of performance measures to track over time.
- *Service-comparison performance evaluation*: this design compares the performance of comparable services and departments in relation to the criteria of performance against which the service is to be evaluated.

Value criteria

In applying these designs it is useful to consider these value criteria, for which data could be gathered to assess performance, relating to inputs, process and outcomes:

- *Consumer quality*: whether the programme gives individuals and the community what they say they want to help them prevent illness and improve health (as measured by people's satisfaction with health promotion and health education programmes).
- *Professional quality*: whether the programme meets individual and community needs for health promotion, as assessed by health promotion professionals, and, whether the programme is designed and provided in a way that professionals believe will prevent illness and promote health (as measured by different professional assessments of the programme, and by outcome indicators and long-term measures).
- *Management quality*: whether the programme is planned, designed and provided or implemented in a way that makes the best use of resources, without waste or mistakes, and that meets higher-level requirements (as measured by the cost of poor quality, and in relation to policies and targets set by higher levels).

Quality in planning and designing health promotion programmes also means that there should be some means of recognizing conflicts between the community views, the professional assessments of needs, and the higher-level requirements, as well as methods for reconciling conflicts and explaining and justifying the final choices. The definition above seeks a balance between the consumer dimension and the professional dimension to quality, between the process and outcome dimensions and also includes the managerial dimension by including cost considerations and higher-level directives.

Evaluating coordination in interventions to population health

One final consideration in evaluation is how activities are coordinated, especially when the programme or service involves enabling a multi-sectorial approach: this is a dimension of the process that may need to be evaluated.

Many health promotion programme and public health services require the involvement of a variety of agencies, interest groups and professionals to improve the population's health. Two aspects to evaluation could be the activities and their success in achieving involvement, and, second, the activities and their success in coordinating agencies.

The following paragraph concentrates on evaluating the second and perhaps easier issue of coordination, once involvement is secured, but recognizes that involvement and coordination issues overlap, and that the involvement of different parties and their roles will change over time.

Cooperation in health promotion can be defined as 'aligning and combining plans and actions for health promotion to reduce preventable mortality and morbidity'. The added value of cooperation and coordination is that the results (e.g. in lower numbers of deaths and morbidity) are greater than the sum of the results of the action of each agency without coordination. For example, employers publicizing the benefits of screening and making provision for access and time off work for screening, where this is coordinated to coincide with publicity promotion by the local authority and local press, as well as with primary and secondary care programmes, and with extra resources supplied to meet the expected demand. The methods and activities used to achieve coordination are often an important aspect to evaluate. Implementation of a health promotion programme depends in part on decisions being made collectively at different levels, which then set the context for decisions at the lower levels. It also depends on involving the right organizations and people in agreeing on the decisions at each level.

Summary

The following is a simple checklist for evaluating a public health service or other types of population health promotion or education programmes.

1 Description of the service, noting any divergence from proposals or plans for the service.
2 Achievement of objectives: To what extent were the objectives achieved?
3 Outcomes: What difference did the programme make to the users or beneficiaries and to different stakeholders?
4 Relevance and appropriateness: Were the activities relevant to changing needs and were they technically and culturally appropriate?
5 Efficiency: How many resources were put in (time and money)? Was there any avoidable waste? Could more outputs have been achieved with the resource inputs? Would a small extra amount of resources have produced disproportionately larger benefits (marginal input benefits)? What were the opportunity costs?
6 Sustainability: With and without continued finance? What are the risks and what are the strengths?
7 Management of the programme: Did the management follow the programme planning and operation requirements? Assess the management performance.

Conclusion

Interventions to populations and communities are different from interventions to health systems or for individual patients. It is true that in such programmes there are interventions directed at individuals. But evaluations also need to consider whether there are also other interventions to health services or other entities that can create conditions which will influence individuals' health behaviour or health-related environments. This chapter has described modifications to designs used to evaluate interventions to populations or communities. It discussed the strengths and weakness of an evaluation of a community programme to prevent heart disease. It also considered ways to evaluate the performance of a public health service.

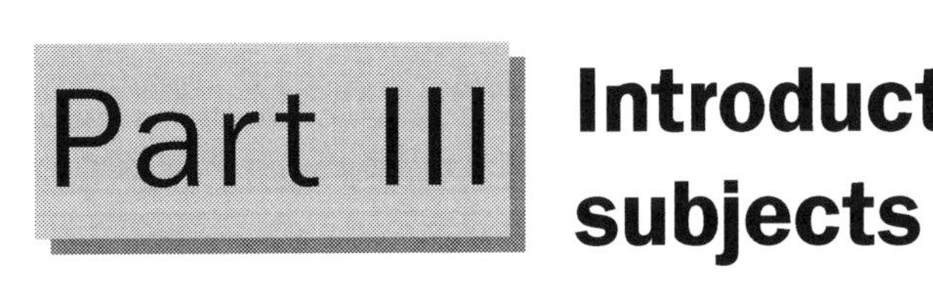

Part III Introduction: Evaluation subjects

Methods to enable change, the digital revolution and money

Part III is where the book looks in more detail about three important subjects: methods for enabling others to change what they do, the digital revolution and money.

Evaluation does not change anything. Implementation does. But we can evaluate an implementation approach and find out if it is effective for making a change. This is what Chapter 10 describes: ways to evaluate implementation approaches, and it explains what an 'implementation approach' is. Usually it is more than telling people 'just do it'.

It's been a long time coming, but the digital revolution is arriving and arriving too fast for evaluators to catch up. There are safety and equity issues with many digital services and we know little about the harm as well as the benefits they can bring – many are unregulated, but also change significantly every few months. Chapter 11 considers how to evaluate digital services and devices, and discusses the modifications to our evaluation methods and the innovation in our evaluation designs that we need to make.

Digital services and devices are one type of complex intervention. But they are also complex social interventions, in that people individually and in groups choose how to use them. This makes the outcomes of a digital intervention less predictable than the outcomes of a drug or surgery on the human body. Chapter 12 looks at what adding 'social' to 'complex intervention' means for evaluation and for the certainty we can have about the local outcomes of a change which may be effective elsewhere.

Money is the subject of Chapters 13 and 14 – or rather the use of resources, which are usually finite. To have relevance to people working in healthcare and health, evaluations need to be able to say something to finish the sentence 'the resource implications of this study are . . .' Chapter 13 shows a simple way to make estimations – it is absolutely not about health economics. It is about estimating return on investment and budget impact analysis. Do economists know only the cost of everything and the value of nothing? Chapter 14 says more about traditional health economic evaluations and the choices they help to inform.

10 Evaluating implementation

Introduction

Evaluation shows us that giving antibiotics one hour before surgery is effective for reducing post-surgical infections. But do all patients who could benefit get the new effective treatment? There are other examples where there is compelling evidence of a more effective intervention, but people do not implement the new better way even when it is less expensive and saves time.

It is not easy to enable professionals or managers to take up new practices or to change their organization, even when the evidence of the effectiveness of these changes is conclusive. In your own life, how much have you changed your own behaviour to implement new knowledge about smoking, diet, exercise or in response to 'doctor's orders'? Implementation of research is perhaps even more challenging for patients, or soon-to-be patients.

Implementation research has grown in recent years because of the challenges in changing practice and organizations to adopt proven improvements in treatments, service delivery models and ways of working. The field draws on change management, behaviour change and other theories and disciplines which examine individual, organizational and social change. It is distinctive in its purpose, which is to understand and enable people and organizations to adopt proven or promising practices and methods in health and welfare organizations. Evaluation of implementation in healthcare and health is a large part of this developing multidiscipline.

But is the intervention – be it a treatment or service delivery model – different from its implementation, which is what is implied above? Surely implementation is part of an intervention? These are two questions that the chapter answers. It considers evaluations of whether an intervention has been copied exactly (fidelity-implementation evaluations). It also considers implementation evaluations of interventions which should not be copied in their content, but which need to be adapted to the setting. These are 'implementation-adaption evaluations'. One type evaluates the continuous adaption people carry out in implementation over time (iterative implementation). Another type evaluates a one-time adaption to the intervention made by the implementers before the implementation (one-time adaption implementation). The latter is an evaluation of how well the implementers adjusted the intervention to the subject or setting, often in their planning and before implementation starts.

What is implementation and is it different from the intervention?

It is true that when we evaluate an intervention, we also evaluate its implementation – how else could you find out if it had any effects? You need to be sure it is fully implemented before assessing outcomes, otherwise it is not a fair evaluation.

When some interventions are evaluated using experimental methods, great efforts are made to ensure that it is fully implemented, so as then to be able to assess whether it is effective. The aim is to increase the internal validity of the study so as to increase the certainty that the outcomes are attributable to the intervention. One way is to rule out, in the case of little effect, the possible explanation that this was due to poor implementation: practitioners did not give the treatment properly or patients did not follow the treatment or the organization did not adopt all the elements of the new practice or service delivery model.

In such studies, more could be done to describe and communicate the implementation methods, for example, how did they ensure patients, providers or organizations were properly exposed to the intervention? One reason to do so is to give others the information to decide if they could repeat it – do we have the resources and conditions which they had in the study evaluation?

Two types of implementation study

One of the issues in designing an implementation evaluation is to decide how many of the intermediate or ultimate outcomes to evaluate. Strictly speaking, implementation evaluations do not consider the full causal chain of outcomes.

One type of implementation study is as part of an outcome or effectiveness evaluation. The implementation study describes what was done to implement the intervention. For example, a Norwegian controlled trial (the outcome study) evaluated the effect of a programme to reduce inappropriate prescribing of antibiotics in primary care practices (Flottorp et al. 2003). A separate process evaluation documented features of the different primary care centres, and of how the programme was implemented in each. The study was then able to explain the large variations in results found in the trial (Flottorp et al. 2003). This explanation would not have been possible without this implementation evaluation.

Often this is a sub-study of an outcome evaluation, but it can be an independent study sometimes called a parallel process evaluation. This is not just to check the outcome evaluation study protocol was applied and the intervention was implemented, which most outcome evaluations do as an integral part of the study. Rather, the purpose is to give details to others, so they can judge if they could do it. The implementation sub-study describes details of what was done to ensure implementation and exposure to the intervention and the conditions which may have been important to help implementation. Such an implementation evaluation addresses the external validity of the study – its generalizability – but in a limited way by providing some information in order to judge whether the same results might be expected elsewhere.

A second type is a cross-site or cross-subject (target) implementation evaluation. This is where effectiveness is proved, but the evaluation concentrates on how it was implemented in one or more sites, or with different patients. The evaluation is of the effectiveness of the implementation methods, and on whether the proven intervention is reproduced in the one or more implementations of it. Examples are some of the studies of the US Veterans' Health Administration (VA) scale-up or spread of proven practices in different VA sites or regions (e.g. Goetz et al. 2008).

This type of implementation evaluation provides a full 'external validity study' because it applies the intervention in settings or populations different to the initial outcome evaluation study-site or sites (Green and Glasgow 2006). This would be where it is thought there may be different outcomes to that found in the effectiveness study site or sites. The aim is to find out if the outcomes are achieved elsewhere with the same intervention. Note that there are also combined evaluations which include both the types described above. These are where an intervention of uncertain effectiveness is evaluated in many different settings.

Some useful definitions

- *Implementation*: enabling people to take up a new way of working which is proved or promises to be more effective. Broadly defined, implementation also includes what is done to enable patients to take up a treatment, behaviour or lifestyle change, as well as the spread or scale-up of proven or promising interventions.
- *Intervention content*: the features of a drug, care practice, service delivery model or policy which is critical to producing desired outcomes, and which are sometimes called 'the active ingredients'. Implementation is to enable people to take up the 'active feature' of the intervention.
- *Implementation evaluation*: an evaluation of the effectiveness of an approach to implement a proven or promising intervention.
- *Outcome evaluation*: an evaluation of the outcomes of an intervention which has been fully implemented.
- *Implementation approach*: the combination of the following elements used to implement an intervention: structure, strategy, and systems and supports for implementation.
- *Intervention-fidelity evaluation*: an assessment of how well an intervention is copied or is 'true to' the specified intervention.
- *Intervention-adaption evaluation*: an assessment of how well an intervention is adapted to its setting or subjects so as to achieve desired results.
- *Spread or scale-up*: the aim of achieving adoption, in many sites or subjects, of a proven or promising intervention.

- *Sustainability*: whether an intervention can be maintained, or whether results are maintained.

The implementation approach

Few interventions are quickly taken up in healthcare without effort and resources for their implementation. There are some exceptions, such as minimally invasive surgery (Royston et al. 1994). However, implementation research has shown that uptake of proven interventions is slow and variable. Many patients do not receive effective interventions or adopt effective behaviours many years after the research has demonstrated the effectiveness.

Research has also found that implementers use different methods to enable more practitioners and services to adopt proven interventions. These include:

- sending practitioners information in the post ('disseminating literature');
- training or education;
- computer alerts or prompts;
- feedback and comparison of performance;
- financial incentives or penalties;
- supervision or regulation requirements, with consequences for non-compliance;
- activating patients to request proven better practices, treatments or services.

The research shows that only some are effective, but also that these need an 'infrastructure' in order to be carried out: training needs a structure of trainers and a schedule, and a system to help deliver the training. An 'approach' to implementation includes the actions taken and methods used, as well as the structure for organizing the actions, the systems and other supports.

Implementation research shows the barriers, but also the facilitators which enable implementation of different interventions and which strategies can be successful. The following draws on this research to give a framework to guide some of the data-gathering to describe the implementation approach which is to be evaluated.

Describing an implementation approach

Gathering data about the following four elements makes it possible to specify what was done to carry out implementation: these four elements working together are what is to be evaluated in an implementation evaluation:

Structure

- the roles and responsibilities for implementation of individuals and groups;
- the defined relationships between those responsible for implementation;
- if relevant, the organizational and group culture which affects implementation.

Strategy

- the activities undertaken and methods used to enable subjects to take up the intervention to apply it or use it.

Systems

- systematic arrangements which enable take-up of the intervention, such as information technology systems, data collection and feedback systems.

Supports

- as an innovative or change-ready culture.

An example of a large-scale structure, strategy and supports is the former Finnish programme for improving prescribing in primary care practice. This involved the formation of a special state agency 'Rhotu', with a national network of primary care 'facilitators' and education programmes and materials (Øvretveit and Mäntyranta 2007).

The above elements have been found to be necessary for effective implementation. By gathering data about each, the evaluation can describe the most important elements in the implementation approach and can characterize and compare approaches. The next question is how to assess the effectiveness of the implementation approach and which data to collect to assess this. One way is to clarify the objectives of implementation and gather data on to what extent these were achieved. For example, whether or how much different patients or providers changed their behaviour or organization to adopt the intervention.

Another is to compare the intervention implemented with the proven version or with what was planned, using an audit evaluation design. A further way is to compare two or more implementations of the intervention and then assess which was more successful, using different data to assess this.

Intervention-fidelity evaluation

If appropriate patients take the medication as directed, then outcomes could be expected similar to those found in similar patients in an earlier trial. But often patients do not follow doctor's orders and also the medication may be inappropriately prescribed for the particular patient. Fidelity of implementation for a drug treatment would be whether properly compounded medications are appropriately prescribed and taken by patients. A fidelity evaluation would assess all these things. One design is the audit design described in Chapter 4, where what is done, is compared to what is specified or with what is planned.

Fidelity means 'true to'. Was the intervention implemented in a way which was 'true to' the intervention which was previously reported to be effective? For example, if patients at risk of stroke are prescribed and take anti-coagulants (blood thinners), then stroke (and heart attack) can be prevented, but blood tests are needed also to reduce the risk of haemorrhage which can occur with anti-coagulants. For full patient benefit, assessing, prescribing and monitoring needs to be carried out exactly, following guidelines based on research. The intervention can be specified in quite some detail and the fidelity of its implementation assessed against this specification.

Evaluating the fidelity of implementation of a model of service delivery such as team-based care, or a disease management model can be more challenging. Perhaps even more difficult is assessing the fidelity of implementation of a multi-component and multi-level health promotion programme. In part, this is because it may not be clear whether some features of the intervention should be adapted and how, and then how to assess if the adaption is effective: evaluation of adaptive implementations is discussed in the next section of this chapter.

The RE-AIM method

One method of evaluating implementation fidelity is the RE-AIM method, which has been used to assess how well different health promotion and other non-drug interventions are implemented. RE-AIM stands for:

- **R**each (proportion of subjects or target population that participated in the intervention).
- **E**fficacy (positive outcomes minus negative outcomes or the success rate if implemented as in the guidelines).
- **A**doption (proportion of settings, practices, and plans that will adopt this intervention).
- **I**mplementation (extent to which the intervention is implemented as intended in the real world).
- **M**aintenance (extent to which a programme is sustained over time).

One example of the use of the RE-AIM is in evaluation of a pharmacy alert intervention. This was to detect and correct medication prescribing errors for all patients who were prescribed medications in a large health system (Magid et al. 2004).

- Reach was assessed by calculating the participation rate and evaluating the degree to which the patients enrolled in the study are representative of the larger patient population (i.e. the 'representativeness' of the sample).
- Effectiveness is assessed across multiple dimensions. Medication errors are the primary outcome. Other outcomes include prescriber, pharmacist, and patient satisfaction; measures of unintended consequences (e.g. false-positive alerts), and potential negative impacts (e.g. repeat patient visits to the pharmacy).
- Adoption is measured by calculating the participation rates of the pharmacies and pharmacists approached to participate in the project. Representativeness of these is assessed by comparing the characteristics of pharmacies and pharmacists that participate to those that do not.

- Implementation is assessed as the degree to which intervention components are delivered as intended. Measures of technical performance include the validity of alerts and system reliability. Measures of pharmacist performance include completeness of progress documentation and adherence to alert recommendations.
- Maintenance is assessed as the sustainability of the intervention's impact during the study (at three, six, nine, and 12 months) and at one year after its completion.

Note that 'adoption', as opposed to 'adaption', in some studies refers to the completed take-up and implementation of an intervention. In other studies, it refers only to the decision to implement an intervention before anything else is done.

An intervention-adaption evaluation

Sometimes infidelity is necessary for good outcomes. Before my girlfriend quotes me on this, I need to explain: infidelity to the intervention. For example, a programme to screen white, urban, professional women for cancer may have proved successful in one city area. However, it may need to be adapted to be culturally appropriate for another ethnic group or in a rural area. Some of the elements may remain the same, such as the technical method for screening. But others may need to be changed, such as some of the contents of the education materials or the language.

There may be a method which has been found to be effective in adapting the intervention to the subjects or setting, for example, getting feedback from different ethnic groups about the education material and revising the material to be more appropriate. If an implementation did not do this, then the intervention might be less effective. In this instance – where there is a proven method for adaption – then we can talk about a type of fidelity evaluation which assesses how well the implementation used the method to adapt the intervention. However, the term fidelity evaluation is more often used to refer to how well the intervention content is copied, not how well the method for adaption is copied.

Continuous or one-time adaption

One type of adaption evaluation is to evaluate the continuous adaption carried out by people when they implement an intervention over time (iterative-adaption implementation). Another type evaluates a one-time adaption to the intervention, made by the implementers before the implementation (one-time adaption implementation). This is an evaluation of how well the implementers adjusted the intervention to the subject or setting, often in their planning and before implementation starts.

A key point is that, if the intervention is known to be effective if it is implemented with fidelity, then the evaluation does not need to assess its impact on patients: the original studies will have assessed and proved this. Rather, the study is of implementation fidelity and possibly of intermediate outcomes, such as changes to processes or percentage of providers complying with the requirements.

However, if some adaption is allowed or needed, then the implementation evaluation not only needs to describe the modification, it also needs to evaluate the effectiveness of the modification in that local setting, as if were a new and unevaluated intervention rather than the implementation of a proven one. This may mean evaluating not only intermediate outcomes, but also the ultimate outcomes to patients.

Other types of implementation evaluation

Implementation' is often viewed as a one-way translation of a proven treatment, test or service model into routine healthcare. The field of knowledge mobilization takes a wider view and considers how knowledge, broadly defined, is found and used by practising individuals and organizations, as well as how they contribute to the knowledge through their experiences and research. 'Collaboration' rather than 'transfer' is the term more often used. Examples of evaluations of knowledge mobilization are evaluations of the different collaborations between UK universities and the NHS services in collaborations for leadership in applied health research and care (CLAHRC) (Rycroft-Malone et al. 2011) and evaluations of some of the Canadian Health Services Research Foundation-funded collaborations (e.g. ARCH 2014).

The interventions to increase knowledge mobilization are of many different types and have different objectives. There are also different users of these evaluations and different purposes for the evaluations. The evaluation design and method will depend on the user, the purpose of the evaluation and the type of intervention and its purpose.

Evaluating spread or scale-up

Spread or scale-up describes what is done to enable many more people and organizations to adopt and put into practice a proven or promising intervention or change. It is implementation on a large scale. As such, scale-up evaluation methods and principles are essentially the same as those already discussed for evaluating implementation.

However, because the scope of the evaluation, in terms of sites covered, is large, data collection tends to rely more on already-reported data or indicators and less on direct data-gathering by the observers visiting sites. Sites may be asked to report data for the evaluation, but with large programmes this may not be feasible. Because of the large amounts of data and the time periods over which the scale-up is to be tracked, visual display of data is increasingly being used, ideally by using geographic displays showing scale-up progress for different areas at different times.

The term scale-up tends to be used more in medical innovation, industry and international health, to describe what is done to enable many practitioners or services in a region to start using a new treatment, practice or service delivery model. For example, the GAVI programme uses different approaches to scale up methods to provide immunization for children in developing countries. Their model for monitoring and evaluating their programmes gives an example of a framework, and one similar to many others, for gathering data about the different aspects and results of a programme (Figure 10.1).

As with all implementation evaluations, an evaluation may be limited to assessing the extent to which inputs, processes and outputs of the model are achieved in a scale-up. However, if there is some uncertainty that outputs will lead to outcomes and impact, and there is time and money for the evaluation, then a limited implementation evaluation may be extended to also assess outcomes and impact.

Useful references for evaluating the scale-up of international health programmes and practices are guides by Adamou (2013) and Brycea et al. (2010). The latter proposes that one way to evaluate the effectiveness of scale-up implementation is to collect indicators of effects in a beneficiary population, including intervention coverage, behaviour change and whether service responsiveness to population needs has increased.

Some studies give good examples for evaluating the scale-up of quality improvement practices and projects: further guidance can be found in Norton et al. (2012), and Øvretveit (2011a, 2011b). Øvretveit (2011b) gives a checklist for an audit design for an evaluation of the scale-up of a quality improvement.

Guidance: evaluating the effectiveness of an implementation approach

Are these implementations different in a way which would require a significantly different evaluation design to evaluate each, even if the evaluation user had the same question, 'Is the implementation effective?'

- an evaluation of the implementation of a training programme which aims to enable nurses in one hospital to use proven methods to reduce pressure ulcers or patient falls;
- an evaluation of the national implementation of clinical guidelines for identifying and caring for depression in older people in primary care;
- an evaluation of the implementation of an electronic medical record system in a regional health system.

Which design is best for evaluating how each intervention is implemented? There is no detailed guidance which can be given, but the following notes some important considerations in choosing an evaluation design:

- *Type of change to be implemented*: a single simple change (a particular treatment, guideline, service delivery model, or service organization to be implemented) or a complex multi-change possibly to a number of levels of the health system, or a continuous change.
- *User actions to be informed*: The evaluation user's actions which the evaluation could inform.

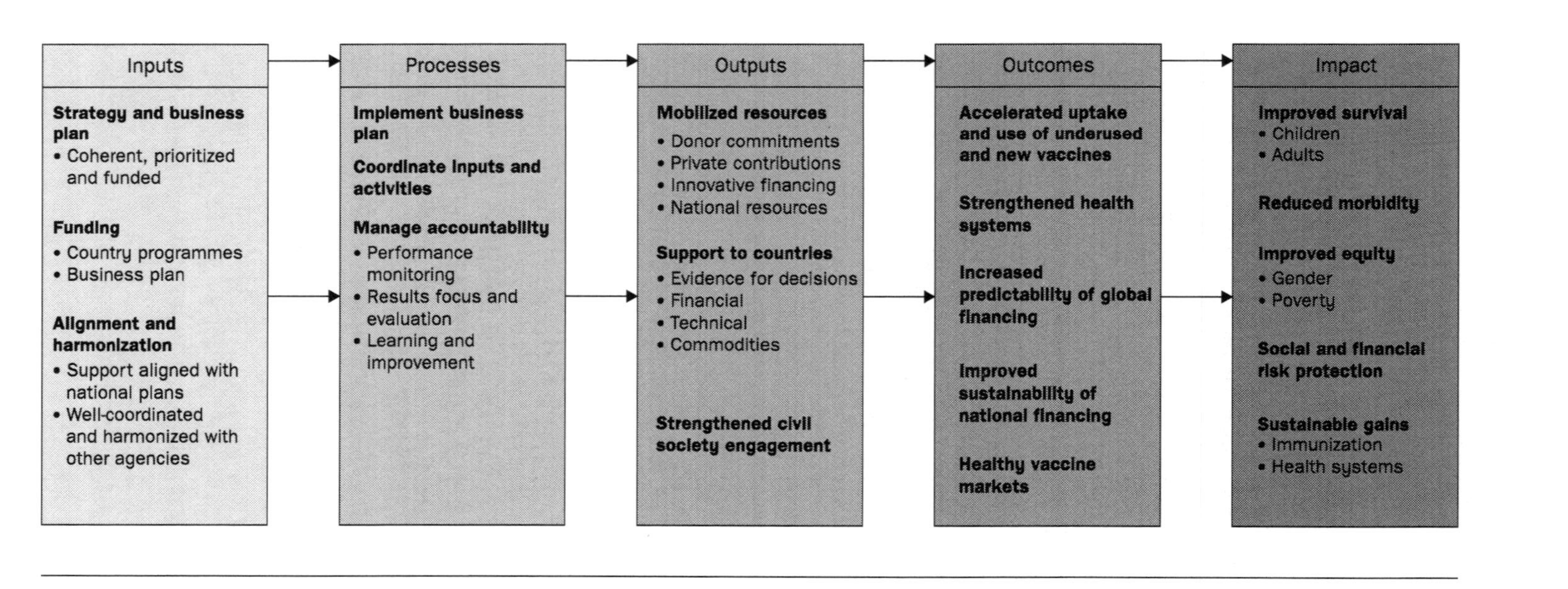

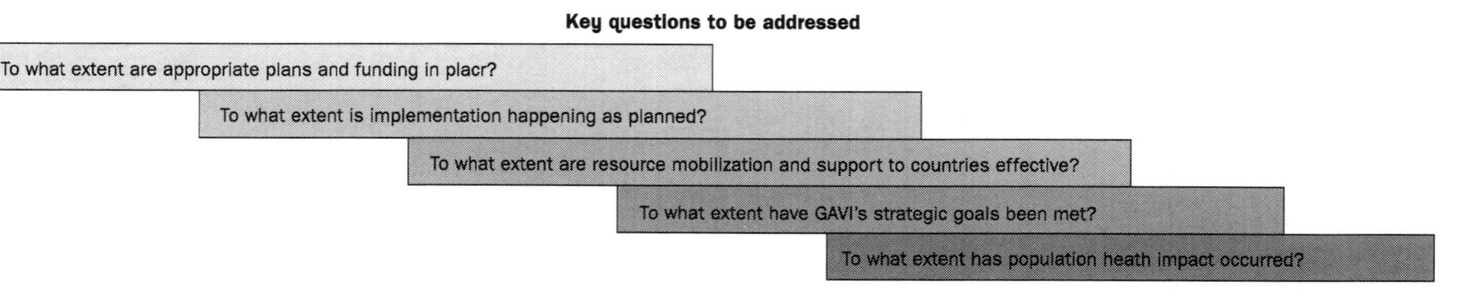

Figure 10.1 The GAVI 2011 model for monitoring and evaluation of scale-up and other programmes

- *Level of the health system*: which level are the implementation actions intended to influence (clinical practitioners, small organizational provider units, provider organizations, health systems, providers in regions or nations)?
- *Implementation only*: is the question only about the approach to implementation, or are there also questions about intermediate and ultimate outcomes – will it need to include an outcome evaluation?
- *Effectiveness or explanatory evaluation*: how much the evaluation is to be limited to effectiveness assessment or broaden into explanatory evaluation (why was this implementation approach successful or less successful?).
- *Action or isolated evaluation*: whether the evaluators are to help the implementation by giving emerging findings from the evaluation to the implementers (action evaluation), or whether the evaluators aim to minimize their influence on the implementation (isolated evaluation).

The implementation evaluation design could also use some or all of these criteria for assessing the extent of the implementation of a change.

Planning and predictions

1 A change plan exists, but no action has been started.
2 Action has been started to make the change, but no change in intermediate or ultimate outcomes has been detected.
3 Action has been started, and a selection of informed observers judge that a change in intermediate or ultimate outcomes is likely.

Implementation correspondence to plan

4 The extent to which the implementation actions taken follow the plan (rate 0–5).
5 Divergence from plan and adjustment was justified and likely to improve implementation.

Breadth of change

6 Change has been documented in a limited sample/area (data: subjective assessment or objective effect measures which can be linked to the change action).
7 Change has been documented in all targeted patients/units/areas (data: subjective assessment or objective effect measures which can be linked to the change action).

Depth of change

8 How deep and extensive has the intended change been to the subjects which have shown some change (rate 0–5) (data: subjective assessment or objective effect measures which can be linked to the change action)?

Maintenance of change

9 A selection of informed observers judge that the change documented in intermediate or ultimate outcomes is likely to remain two years after.
10 A follow-up shows evidence that the change documented in intermediate or ultimate outcomes remains two years after.

There are also criteria for assessing the contribution of research to implementation of a change. These are:

1 Actions the researchers took to influence the change was documented (rate 0–5).
2 An assessment was made by the researchers of how much their actions contributed to the change, including a consideration of the other influences on the change.
3 The strength of evidence that the change was caused by the research, or the likely percentage contribution of the research to the change relative to other influences causing the change.

Conclusion

Evaluation may show an intervention is effective, but this, in itself, does not change anything. Research has found that more people dispute evaluation findings when these conflict with their interests, or have reasons not to adopt it when the science is good. Different implementation approaches have been developed to enable people to change to the new better way, be it in professional practice, service organization or in patient lifestyle. Are there effective ways to implement proven interventions so that more patients benefit more quickly from research discoveries, where evidence is compelling?

This chapter considered how we evaluate 'implementation approaches'. It defined implementation as what is done to enable people to take up a new better way. It showed how to describe and distinguish one implementation approach from others by describing the structure used for implementation, the strategy of actions and methods, and the supports such as information systems.

Fidelity evaluation assesses whether the intervention is implemented in a way that reproduces the key features which produced better outcomes elsewhere. But some interventions need to be adapted to different situations: intervention-adaption evaluations assess how well the implementers have continually adapted the intervention to the situation. Such evaluations may need to assess whether the adapted intervention is effective in producing ultimate outcomes, as well as assessing implementation.

Generally, we know more about which interventions are effective than about how to make them used in healthcare and by patients. Implementation evaluation can define the different strategies and show which is most effective for a particular intervention. This can contribute to making it possible for more people more quickly to benefit from medical discoveries, service delivery models and public health programmes which have been proved effective. It can contribute to reducing disparities in the provision and uptake of effective treatments and services.

11 Evaluating digital health technologies

Introduction

Digital technologies made a slow start in health, but their use will accelerate rapidly. Can they be designed and applied to enhance rather than diminish human dignity and well-being? Can we use them to bring out what we value most in the best caring and service encounters? Evaluation can help shape these technologies to fulfil important values in healthcare, and can check that they do not bring harm to patients or providers by clumsy design and implementation.

Digital health technologies (DHTs), which include the internet, are becoming a part of most health services and are increasingly being used by patients and citizens. But how much do different technologies really contribute to improving healthcare and health? Evaluation can help answer this and other questions raised by different stakeholders. Evaluation of implementation of these technologies is especially important, given that many have been costly failures, and poor implementation causes harm to patients. This was demonstrated in Chapter 8, which discussed the design of an evaluation of the implementation of a shared summary care record in the UK (Greenhalgh and Russell 2010; Greenhalgh et al. 2010b).

Evaluations of DHTs may require different designs and approaches to those commonly used to evaluate other health interventions, even though many principles for assessing value are similar. The aim of this chapter is to give an overview of these designs, and about when each is most useful.

What are DHTs?

DHT is a term broader than health information technology (HIT). HIT typically covers systems for data-gathering and data provision such as electronic medical records as well as health websites and services. In addition to these, DHTs include devices with digital elements, such as an automatic IV infusion device; which might not transmit information, or a mobile ultrasound.

Types of DHTs

One example of a DHT is an electronic medical record (EMR), another is a movement sensor alert system. Would a different approach be used to evaluate the implementation of an electronic medical record in a small primary healthcare centre, to the approach for evaluating the effectiveness of a movement sensor alert system for older people in their homes?

One answer is that it depends on what you mean by an 'approach' and this will be considered below. Some things about the evaluation of these two DHTs would be different and some might be the same. The following categorizes some types of DHT in terms of the likelihood of DHTs within one category requiring significantly different 'approaches' for their evaluation – it does not cover all DHTs, but aims to highlight the need to consider the type of DHT in deciding which criteria by which to evaluate it and which methods to use for the evaluation.

Individual documentation DHTs

This family includes systems for documenting non-medical data about an individual patient, as well as medical data documentation systems such as EMRs, EHRs and ePHRs.

Computer decision support (CDS) systems

'Pop-up' suggestions giving reminders or alerts are the visible output of one type of CDS system and often work from within an electronic medical record when it is opened for a patient or at log-in by the clinician. There are many other types of CDS system, such as an expert guidance system for giving advice for patients who call into an information service. All obviously require a computer system to be operating, and usually they are 'implemented into' an existing system. One of the evaluation criteria is how well they can be implemented in different places and systems, and others are the cost of doing so and how well the CDS system works within the system.

'Remote DHT systems'

This category includes telemedicine for provider to patient or provider to another provider. Telemonitoring typically uses devices in the home to pick up and transmit data. Note that the latter typically involve a care manager who will respond to alerts – a number of DHTs are combined with staffed services, or are one element of a larger improvement, which can make the evaluation of the DHT on its own difficult.

Websites

Some websites may be for information only, or enable the user to interact through the site with others. Standards for assessing websites have been developed (HONF 2013).

Digital devices for health services

These include bar-code readers, drug-dispensing equipment, portable ultrasound, ECG for smart phone, and nano sensors which detect endothelial cells before a heart attack, as well as digitally enabled surgical equipment. Health technology assessment methods which emphasize safety can be used to assess these.

Management and population health DHT systems

These include systems for performance and operations management, such as scenario or workflow simulations; simulations to help design; radio-frequency identification (RFID) for flow tracking; management information systems (costing, resource utilization); systems to analyse clinical information databases/clinical registries and systems for public and population health and planning such as health geo-mapping.

Why should we evaluate DHTs?

- To find independent evidence of effectiveness: pilot experiences are often reported by enthusiasts in well-resourced settings and might not be repeated in other settings and patient groups. There is a positive reporting and technology bias.
- To assess whether the costs are worth the benefits, especially the costs of implementation and maintenance.
- To assess risks of unexpected harm or safety risks of poor implementation.
- To find the differential impact on social groups and if disadvantaged groups are less able to benefit from the use of DHTs and if DHTs increase inequalities.
- To contribute to the improvement of the DHT, for example, in user-interface design.

Box 11.1 An evaluation of a DHT: example 1

Researchers in Sweden evaluated a specific type of computer-supported service which allowed physician and patient together to review the history of treatment and its changing effect on the patients' disability (rheumatoid arthritis).

The DHT was a clinical database, a computer terminal which allowed the patient to enter their current pain scores for different bone joints, and a computer display which could show graphically the current disability score, as well as previous treatments and disability scores on the same screen. It also included software which input the data into the database and calculated and graphically displayed the time trends.

Patients and providers were asked how satisfied they were with the system, implicitly comparing it to the visit and consultations before the system was introduced to the clinic. In the patient questionnaire, 96 per cent of patients (n = 44) rated their impression of the system as 'excellent to good'. Interviews with both patients and providers (n = 6) indicated that both were very positive about the patient overview which the system gave which displayed data previous to the clinical encounter.

The researchers summarized the interview findings as showing that the system 'enabled patient involvement through engagement, education, and communication with the provider, who appreciated them as time-saving for managing data and as decision support' (Hvitfeld et al. 2009).

The example in Box 11.1 illustrates a number of points important for all DHT evaluations:

- *Describe the DHT*: a description of 'the item' to be evaluated is necessary in order that the reader can understand what the findings are referring to: if outcomes are reported, then reader needs to know 'what do these come out of?' and possibly also 'could I implement this?'. The term 'intervention' is often used to describe 'the item' evaluated.
- *Separate the DHT*: it is always difficult to separate the item from its surroundings (the 'context') in order to evaluate only 'the item', and sometimes it is inappropriate to do so.
- *DHT–service combinations*: often evaluations are not of the DHT alone but are of a combination of the DHT and the service and of how the DHT was integrated into a particular service or formed part of a new service redesign. The evaluation may be more of the service redesign than of the DHT per se. For example, an evaluation of an EMR is usually an evaluation of an EMR operating in a particular clinic or hospital. EMRs can be evaluated in a laboratory in relation to certain performance criteria, but most DHTs are evaluated in real-life situations. Some of the negative findings about telemedicine in the largest evaluation to date may be due more to the different 'whole system transformations' they were part of in different sites rather than the DHT system itself (Cartwright et al. 2013).
- *What is not evaluated*: the evaluation did not report the costs of introducing the system, or the benefits of using it to compare physicians' performance. It did not consider safety risks (which include data security), how well it was implemented, the conditions needed to implement it, and only considered the two general value criteria of patient and provider satisfaction.
- *Prove attribution*: the evaluation has to establish that the primary cause of the outcomes is the DHT which was evaluated, and not caused by something else. The example assumes that those surveyed and interviewed were referring to the system which was being evaluated by their replies. The 'attribution challenge' is how the evaluator establishes that any so-called outcomes are in fact outcomes of the item being evaluated and not something else. Might the replies be referring to more than just 'the new system'?

- *Assess generalization*: could someone else introduce this DHT and, if they did, would they observe similar results in terms of the satisfaction of both the patient and the provider? The 'generalization challenge' is how the evaluator assesses and communicates what would be necessary to implement a similar DHT elsewhere, and whether similar outcomes could be expected.

What does 'evaluating a DHT' mean?

Evaluating a DHT means judging its value for a particular person or evaluation user group according to the criteria they want to use. The 'evaluation criteria' represent what is important to them when making a decision which is to be informed by the evaluation. Examples are: How much does it cost? Will it save time or need more time to use it? Does it increase or reduce risks of harm? These are three questions implying criteria by which a user will judge the value of a DHT.

Evaluating a DHT is judging the value of the DHT, by gathering information about it in a systematic way, and by making a comparison, for the purpose of making a better informed decision about the DHT.

User-focused evaluation

One approach to evaluation is to take an evaluation user focus (not necessarily the user of the DHT), which is the approach taken by this chapter. This does not mean that criteria other than those important to the user of the evaluation cannot be included by the evaluator, but it does emphasize the need to discover in dialogue with the user of the evaluation which criteria they use to judge the DHT and which decisions they want to be informed by the evaluation (Øvretveit 1998, 2002).

Types of evaluation according to the comparison made

The comparison made in Box 11.1 was with how the clinic worked before the DHT was introduced: the patients and providers were asked to give their perceptions of the system, and implicitly to compare it with what had happened before. 'Before' and 'after' comparison is one of four ways to judge value by comparison. The comparison can be:

- comparing before with after the introduction of the DHT ('effect' or 'outcome' evaluation as in Box 11.1);
- comparing the DHT with nothing, or with some comparable thing;
- comparing whether the planned objectives are achieved ('objectives achievement evaluation');
- comparing the implementation of the DHT with what was planned as one way to judge the value of the implementation (implementation evaluation).

Evaluations of DHTs are always limited: there is only limited time and money to gather a limited amount of data so we have to focus on gathering data about the three subjects which are important:

- what is the DHT which was actually implemented (the description of the intervention)?
- the few criteria we are going to use to judge value (e.g. outcomes for patients, provider satisfaction, costs, risks of harm);
- the context, if there is no controlled comparison which seeks to rule out the role of context.

What is special about evaluating DHTs?

One thing which makes DHTs interesting for evaluators is they often call for new and innovative approaches to their evaluation. For example, some DHTs will be continually changed in a significant way during the evaluation because the technology changes, or will be adapted to the implementation setting or user group. Evaluation methods which are able to describe the changes, why they were made and also provide data about impact are often needed. This calls for different methods than experimental designs which are the dominant evaluation method in medical and health services research, or for innovations in such design.

Debate about appropriate evaluation methods for DHT

This chapter takes the view that the evaluation method which is appropriate is the one which best answers the users' questions for the particular DHT in question. There is a debate within the informatics and DHT evaluation community about 'which methods are most appropriate'. This debate has usefully shown both the strengths and weaknesses of different methods for different DHTs and questions.

Some researchers take the view that controlled experimental trials should be the design of choice, especially for those DHTs where the stakes are high if the DHT were rapidly adopted without rigorous testing – where the potential risks of harm for patients and costs of the intervention are high (Liu and Wyatt 2011). But it is also widely accepted within this field that a range of other evaluation designs are appropriate for answering different questions, and for evaluating those DHTs which do not expose patients, providers or others to risk of harm and are inexpensive (UKIHI 2001; Stoop et al. 2004; Craig et al. 2008; Øvretveit 2013).

Lehmann and Ohno-Machado (2011) note that informatics systems involve multiple interventions, and that 'adherence, in terms of adoption, varies greatly within an institution; and training for HIT systems is notoriously variegated'. They note that the practical challenges of using some controlled trial experimental designs prevent their being used, and that the technology of the intervention is often changed during the trial. Their commentary in the scientific journal, *Journal of American Medical Informatics Association* (JAMIA) notes:

> JAMIA publishes qualitative evaluations and reports of studies that employ methodologies designed to model behavioral and social systems and does not restrict its publications to quantitative evaluations or studies that utilize

> methodologies designed to model physical systems. Therefore, JAMIA ignores the perceived dichotomy between 'soft' versus 'hard' sciences. The field of health and biomedical informatics is diverse and each study is unique; thus, it is important to understand what is most appropriate for a particular investigation and to avoid a priori rule-in or rule-out of particular methodologies.
>
> (Lehmann and Ohno-Machado 2011)

Liu and Wyatt (2011) note some of the criticisms of RCTs in the field of medical informatics:

- Trials are unethical.
- Clinical information systems are too complex to be evaluated by RCTs.
- There is mixed evidence that RCTs can be successfully applied to medical informatics.
- Other study designs can also provide evidence that is just as reliable as RCTs.
- Trials are too expensive.
- Theory or case studies can reliably predict what works.
- Clinical information systems can do no harm.
- RCTs take too long and technology in medical informatics moves too quickly.
- Trials answer questions that are not of interest to medical informatics.

They answer each criticism and present the case for RCTs, arguing that this approach has been under-used in medical informatics, could be used with modifications, and needs to be used when the risk/cost stakes are high. They describe quasi-experimental designs (also discussed in Friedman and Wyatt 2006), and note how a multi-arm randomized trial can be used to quantify the contributions of different components of a complex intervention.

When evaluating DHTs, Friedman et al. (2006) propose that evaluation should assess:

- the extent of the fit between the innovation and the context;
- the stakeholder perceptions and experiences of the innovation;
- the extent of the change to services and outcomes;
- the extent to which new practices have become embedded;
- the effects (and unintended consequences) of the innovation on services, service users and the wider system;
- learning that can be transferred to other settings and how this relates to the broader literature on innovation.

Williams (2011) proposes:

> When measuring inputs and outputs of innovations, the former are likely to include quantifiable financial, human and physical resources alongside the more difficult to measure tacit knowledge. Issues to bear in mind when drawing up a list of outcome measures include not just benefits to the organization and patients, but also the distribution of positive net benefits, for example, between organizations, functions and user groups.

Innovation potential, 'emergent properties' and 'affordance'

Will it encourage new uses and value applications which may be difficult to imagine? This is another feature of some DHTs which may be important to assess – how they encourage, enable or lay the basis for new future uses of benefit to patients or to reduce costs? In Sweden, a DHT clinical database system was developed for physicians and nurses to enter clinical patient data and patient-reported outcomes. The IT infrastructure and the social agreements for the system enabled and encouraged uses which were not originally imagined: patients entering in their data used mobile devices and were reading graphic displays on their mobiles showing the time trends of treatments related to their reported outcomes. Also shown were links to genomic databases for research, and links to hospital statistics to allow cost per patient related to outcomes for each physician and department. Evaluations may need to include in their assessments the 'infrastructure' value of a DHT in what it may enable in the future, as well as whether using the DHT encourages and enables users to discover or invent new uses.

Summary: considerations when adapting traditional evaluation methods to evaluate DHTs

Some evaluation methods are designed for evaluating complex social interventions like DHTs (Øvretveit 2013). Many traditional evaluation methods such as a controlled trial may need modifications or may not be appropriate or feasible:

- Is the DHT going to change in any significant way during the evaluation? Will implementation change the nature of the DHT?
- Is the DHT designed to be tailored to the setting or purpose during implementation such that the implemented DHT will be unique? Could others implement the same DHT or will tailoring always be necessary?
- Does the user of the evaluation want feedback from the evaluation during the implementation to help improve the DHT or its implementation?
- How dependent is the DHT on other technologies in order to be implemented fully?
- What scope does the evaluator have to add valuation criteria and data which the user may not see as top priority?

Who will fund the time and work needed to gather data about whether the DHT disadvantages any social group, or to explore risks, or to assess costs and benefits for different stakeholders, if the evaluation funder is not able to pay for these data and the evaluator considers these to be important, and valuable for publication?

- Can the DHT be conceptualized in a picture ('model') showing its elements, and can the picture show what type of intermediate and later effects might be expected, and features of the surrounding environment which may be important in implementing and sustaining the DHT in operation?
- Would an assessment of readiness for adoption provide some of the data needed by the user? Could such an assessment help explain implementation experience and help provide information for generalization?

Box 11.2 An evaluation of a DHT: example 2

A cluster randomized trial was carried out in the UK with 217 primary care centres randomly allocated to 'telehealth-assisted care' vs. 'normal care' (n = 2600 people with social and medical needs) (Figure 11.1) The telehealth intervention was not standardized and varied between the centres, but all used a pulse oximeter for chronic obstructive pulmonary disease, a glucometer for diabetes, and weighing scales for heart failure patients. Sites asked patients to take clinical readings at the same time each day for up to five days per week.

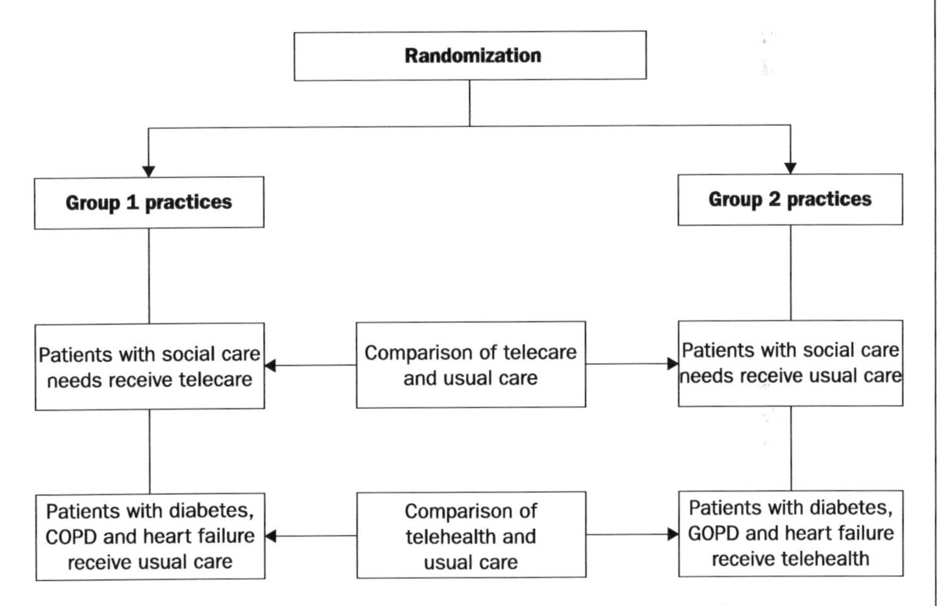

Figure 11.1 Cluster randomization to telehealth-assisted care and normal care

Source: Steventon et al. (2013).

Data were gathered from service statistics (about use of hospital, primary care services and medications). Symptom questions and educational messages were sent to participants either via the telehealth base unit or via a television 'set top box'. At the end of each patient's session, data from clinical readings and symptom questions were transmitted to monitoring centres via a secure server. Monitoring centres were staffed by specialist nurses from local health organizations, who used protocols to respond to the information from patients.

The primary end point was the percentage of patients admitted to hospital over 12 months: 46.8 per cent of the intervention vs. 49.2 per cent controls were admitted. The conclusion was recorded: 'Telecare as implemented in the Whole Systems Demonstrator trial did not lead to significant reductions in service use.'

(Steventon et al. 2013)

Approaches to evaluation

The example in Box 11.2 used 'an approach' to evaluation which was not just the controlled trial design, but involved a experimental perspective with certain assumptions about how to exclude influences other than telehealth on the before/after data which were gathered. In contrast, the first example evaluation was not experimental but 'observational' and involved qualitative data perceptions as data about outcomes: it used a retrospective assessment by DHT users, and they implicitly made a 'before/after' comparison.

Neither example used a model to conceptualize the DHT and effects of interest or used this model to decide which data to collect, or to decide on a planning method to be used, such as a case study or context-sensitive evaluations or implementation evaluations. Some models use a retrospective observational design and others use this within an action-feedback paradigm as opposed to a detached researcher paradigm, gathering both qualitative and quantitative data.

In this chapter, 'an approach' to evaluation is the combination of the following descriptors of types of evaluations.

The evaluation 'paradigm': experimental, observational or action evaluation

- *Experimental*: planning is done to introduce the DHT as if it were an experiment, with data collection before, then it is implemented and data gathered afterwards.
- *Observational*: detached researchers document the DHT as implemented and observe effects of interest.
- *Action-evaluation*: unlike those above, this type of evaluation aims to change the DHT as it is implemented by providing implementers with data gathered from the evaluation, such as users' first experiences with early versions. Often action evaluation is integral to DHT development, for example, for fast iteration of website designs.

The 'model' of the DHT and its effects

This may or may not include features of the 'context' of the DHT implementation and its operation in practice, such as the financing and regulation environment, or the type of setting within which the DHT is introduced.

The design of the evaluation

Design describes the time perspective over which the evaluation data are collected and shows the dates and methods used to collect data, often in a diagram. It also describes whether a comparison is made with no DHT, or with something similar. A flow picture of how patients or providers are selected and allocated to groups shows one type of design.

The data collection and analysis

A model or the design may be used to specify the data to be collected. Collection is broadly described as quantitative (numbers) or qualitative (text record of what a person says or writes down) or combining both (mixed methods') and aims to collect data about the DHT as implemented, about the effects, and sometimes about the implementation (structure for implementation, strategy and support systems for implementation), and sometimes about the context.

Carrying out a DHT evaluation

Although different evaluations will use different methods suited to the purpose of the evaluation, planning and carrying out most types of DHT evaluation can be described in eight steps. The outline below uses the eight-steps approach and describes them in relation to carrying out a DHT evaluation:

1 User goal specification
2 Reviewing relevant research
3 Defining practical and scientific questions
4 Listing and choosing designs
5 Preparing for the evaluation
6 Data-gathering
7 Data analysis
8 Reporting, publishing and dissemination activities.

User goal specification

Before planning the design and gathering the data, the evaluator needs to be clear about who the evaluation is for (the 'user' or 'customer' of the evaluation), and know the user's decisions which the evaluation is intended to inform. The user's goals for the evaluation are the goals of the evaluator. For example: 'I need to know if physicians use the clinical decision support and how much.' Or, 'I need to know if the strategy used by in another region is an effective way for us to implement this.' Evaluations which focus on one category of users, and the key decisions which they want the evaluation to inform, are able to focus their resources, design and data-gathering on one purpose and to be more successful in this purpose. No evaluation can answer all users' questions, and few can answer more than one or two. User goal specification is best carried out by the evaluator discussing and negotiating with representative users or the funder about which decisions the user needs to make that could be informed by the evaluation.

Reviewing relevant research

Step 2 is reviewing the relevant research to find out if the users' questions have already been answered in whole or in part by published research. But this is also to find models or frameworks from others' evaluations in order to conceptualize the DHT and which aspects of its context may be important for its implementation. Reviews can be simple or long and complex and everything in between. How much time is spent on this stage and which methods are used depend on the timescale and resources available.

Defining practical and scientific questions

Step 3 brings the review of previous research together with the users' definition of the purpose of the evaluation to define both the practical and scientific questions to be answered by the evaluation. This stage also involves defining the evaluation parameters: the report target date, the budget and skills available for the research and how much data can be used which has already been collected.

Listing and choosing designs

Step 4 is to list potential designs and make a choice about which will provide acceptable answers within the timescale and with the resources available. Some designs are ruled out by the timescale and the resources available for the evaluation, or by other constraints or practical issues:

- Experimental and quasi-experimental designs are suitable for questions about the effectiveness or outcomes of the DHT.
- Observational designs can be used for both effectiveness and implementation questions.
- Action evaluations may be suitable for questions about how to improve the DHT while it is being implemented.

When considering what outcome data to collect, consider whether accessible data already exists: any special primary data collection by the evaluator is costly in time and money.

Preparing for the evaluation

Once the design has been decided, then step 5 starts, practical arrangements can be planned, using a time-task map about when and how to gather data. This shows who does what, and the steps for any ethical approval which may be needed.

Data-gathering

To answer the evaluation questions, in step 6, data need to be gathered from different sources, using different methods and stored in a way to make analysis easy. Data can be in qualitative or quantitative form and collected using data collection methods which are known to most researchers. Step 7, data analysis, is far easier and quicker if the data, when collected, have been stored in a way which was organized with an eye toward how the data would later be analysed.

Reporting, publishing and dissemination activities

An evaluation of a DHT is only effective when it is used to decide what to do, such as whether or how to change a service, improve the DHT or to spread a change. The findings of the evaluation need to be communicated and available to users at a time when they can use it (step 8).

More details about evaluating DHTs can be found in Poon et al. (2009), Ammenwertha et al. (2004), Eisenstein et al. (2011) and Øvretveit (2013).

Conclusion

There are undoubtedly challenges in evaluating DHTs. Many change while you are evaluating them, depend on careful implementation for their effectiveness and may have effects which are difficult to predict. DHTs call for resourcefulness in applying traditional evaluation methods, and innovation in developing new methods. Their increasing application in healthcare and in people's everyday lives calls for independent assessments of their effects and costs if we are to reap the benefits more quickly, more safely and for all income groups.

12 Evaluating complex social interventions

Introduction

Have you ever done something differently because of what someone said? Or because they promised you money if you did what they said? Other people influence not only what we think but what we do. Many health interventions are people talking to other people to change their behaviour. Interventions to patients by a clinician are not all physical such as surgery or physiotherapy, or chemical such as biological drugs. Most involve education, persuasion or other means to influence behaviour, as part or all of the intervention. Interventions to change clinicians' behaviour also use people-influencing methods, as do interventions to change organizations or policy.

Are there some influencing methods which work better than others? There is a great need for evaluation of the effectiveness of 'people-influencing methods' in changing healthcare or improving health. This chapter describes why these methods can be thought of as complex social interventions. Thinking of them in this way allows us to answer questions other than 'Does it work?', such as 'How would we get the same results in our service?' In this chapter we also consider different proposals for improving evaluations of complex social interventions: (1) apply controlled trials more rigorously (e.g. NYT 2014); (2) apply less rigorous but more relevant methods (Riley et al. 2013); or (3) use theory-informed explanatory observational designs (Øvretveit 2013)

If an evaluation is only to assess if the intervention made a difference in one respect, then why not use the same design which we use to assess outcomes of a drug treatment? If we are just interested in whether, for example, training changed the way physicians prescribed antibiotics, then why not use one of the experimental designs?

This chapter proposes that we can do this, but we can also answer other questions if we consider how people interpret and respond to the intervention. What people think may not be so important for physical and biological interventions, because the causal processes are similar in most people. But for other types of influencing intervention, understanding how people choose to be influenced, help to predict the outcomes in others, apart from those in the study.

The chapter proposes that some evaluations can usefully discover how other influences, apart from the intervention one, affect whether people are influenced by the intervention: if the training to change antibiotic prescribing is done at a time when newspapers also happen to be covering the dangers of over-prescribing, this may affect both patients and clinicians and this, in turn, may cause changes in prescribing and dispensing rates. This influence may be the 'context' or newspaper articles may be stimulated as part of a cluster of actions which are defined as 'the intervention'.

The chapter shows how designs which take into account how people interpret an intervention can be useful for answering transferability or generalization questions such as, 'Would we get the same results here as in the study?' It shows that, for certain questions, interventions are usefully viewed not just as complex interventions (CI) (multi-part or multi-level), but also as complex social interventions (CSI) – that people and groups are involved and what they think affects whether the intervention is effective.

First, what is the difference between a complex intervention and a complex social intervention? Large-scale interventions such as national reforms are clearly complex, but are other interventions also complex, or is it just how we think about them?

Why do we need to evaluate complex social interventions and what are they?

Around the world, substantial amounts of time and money are being spent on large-scale intentional change programmes: schemes to introduce digital health technologies, national, regional- or system-based quality and safety programmes, and programmes to influence performance with financial incentives or indicator-reporting.

In the USA, the progress of the Affordable Care Act health reforms requires that demonstration projects document effective methods to improve quality and control costs (PPACA 2010). The US Center for Medicare and Medicaid Innovation (CMMI) requires timely but also rigorous evaluations of the complex interventions which it is funding (Gold et al. 2011). Smaller-scale changes to one hospital or unit are also complex social interventions, such as:

- 'care bundles' introduced in one intensive care unit (ICU) to reduce ventilator-associated pneumonia (VAP), or central line-associated blood stream infections (CLABSI);
- a multiple intervention to a long-term care facility to prevent patient falls, or to prevent pressure ulcers, or to prevent infections using a hand hygiene programme;
- introducing a computer decision support system to assist physicians in diagnosis and treatment decisions.

What are 'complex interventions'?

Authoritative guidance for medical researchers was published in 2000 describing a complex intervention as being 'built up from a number of components, which may act both independently and inter-dependently' (Medical Research Council 2000). Craig et al. (2008) updated this guidance and describe the following as features of an intervention which make it complex:

- the number of interacting components within the experimental and control interventions;
- the number and difficulty of behaviours required by those delivering or receiving the intervention;
- the number of groups or organizational levels targeted by the intervention;
- the number and variability of outcomes;
- the degree of flexibility or tailoring of the intervention permitted.

Table 12.1 shows increasing degrees of the objective complexity of interventions and their implementation strategies, and the level from which the intervention is initiated. Evaluations are needed of each type of intervention, and will require different evaluation methods to answer different user questions.

What are 'complex *social* interventions'?

There are features of the 'social' part of many interventions which are not fully considered in the above Medical Research Council guidance. We can add value to evaluations by thinking more about the social parts of these complex interventions:

Table 12.1 Different complexity of interventions and level of intervention

Level of intervention	Simple intervention	Complex intervention and progressive implementation (CPI)	Complex intervention and adaptive implementation (CAI)
Region, national (policy, public health)	Intervention: directive to withdraw a pharmaceutical	CLABSI bundle implemented in some ICUs, then more ICUs added	Pilot an Accountable Care Organization, then revise after government funding model is changed, then make further changes
Health system	Change the wound care package we use	Same as above	Infection control programme, continually revised
Health facility	Change the hospital signage, to help patients find different services	Same as above	Infection control programme, continually revised
Team or department	Install more hand-washing gel dispensers	ICUs use CLABSI bundle with some and then all patients	Lean manufacturing principles applied to make initial changes, then more changes after experience with testing first set of changes and with changes in reimbursement

- Care improvement 'bundles' such the combination of actions which need to be taken in an ICU to reduce ventilator-associated pneumonia (VAP) or central line-associated blood stream infections (CLABSI). These can be evaluated as complex interventions to answer questions about efficacy using the designs described in the above guidance (Craig et al. 2008). Or they can be evaluated as complex social interventions.
- Quality and safety improvement initiatives: local small projects or large-scale programmes such as the IHI saving 100,000 lives programme (Berwick et al. 2006).
- The 'CSI' term refers to the intervention being both complex and social. But it also refers to the 'unit of change' such as a group or organization being complex and social. These interventions are often not standardizable, unlike pharmaceutical interventions, and the effects on the unit of change are not as predictable. Evaluation designs which are suited to assessing the effects of a changing intervention to social groups are often necessary to answer the questions of the customers of the evaluation.

Many interventions – such as a care improvement 'bundle' to reduce infections – can be thought of as complex interventions (CIs) or as complex social interventions (CSIs). The distinction is not so much about the intervention, as it is about the way it is conceptualized: the term 'social' points to evaluation methods and questions less familiar in medical and health services research.

Complex

Complexity is both in the nature of the intervention, and in how it is conceptualized by the evaluator: any intervention can be conceptualized as simple (e.g. one action causes results) or as complex (e.g. many parts interacting). The features of complexity which are important for designing an evaluation and data gathering are:

- *Content* of the intervention: it is complex if it involves a number of changes or is 'multiple component' (e.g. a CLABSI bundle).
- *Implementation* may involve an infrastructure of groups, a strategy of actions, and information technology or other systems to support care providers or patients.
- *Change* may be made to the content or implementation at different times. The intervention may be adapted to fit the organization or adapted in response to changes in, for example, financing. Many programmes which are the subject of CSI evaluations are reviewed and revised at certain times, and these changes need to be taken into account in the evaluation. This is especially so when evaluating quality improvement projects where testing and iteration are part of the change methods.
- *Levels* of the health system at which the intervention is directed. The components of the intervention may be directed at a single level, for example, all directed at individual care provider behaviour (e.g. training, reminders and feedback). But some interventions also involve actions to influence more than one level (e.g. in addition, directives or financial incentives to influence management to support the care provider's behaviour in different ways) and to create organizational or wider conditions to enable lower-level change (e.g. state financial incentives or regulations).

Social

'Social', when added to 'complex intervention', highlights the human and group aspects of the change. It draws attention to the behavioural content of the change (e.g. 'wash your hands') and the psychological (choice, motivation) and social nature of the implementation (e.g. project groups, training programmes, negotiating union agreements, negotiating changes to physicians' schedules and work practices).

'Social' implies that the intervention is not acting through predictable physical processes following natural laws, but according to psychological, social and political patterns and influences. These have different 'causal processes', because people individually and in groups have a choice about how they act and influence each other.

This does not mean that there are not discoverable regularities and patterns in human behavior. It does mean that replication and prediction are less precise than it is for many natural physical and biological processes where human interpretation and choice have no or little influence. How one group behaves in one place may be different to how another group behaves elsewhere. Knowing why groups do what they do may help to predict or design an intervention elsewhere.

Intervention

A third set of concepts define the 'intervention', when applied to changes of this type rather than to discrete pharmaceutical or surgical interventions to patients:

- *Scale*: changes falling within the category of 'CSI' can be large, covering many organizations or units or people (e.g. national safety programme) or small covering one unit (e.g. a multiple-component 'CLABSI care bundle' in one ICU).
- *Unit of change*: the people, organizations, facilities or communities which are intended to be different, as a result of the intervention (e.g. a CLABSI intervention aims to change ICU care providers' behaviour and ultimately patient outcomes).
- *Content*: the way in which the units of change are intended to be different after the intervention (e.g. care providers carry out the components of the CLABSI bundle: (1) Wash your hands; (2) Clean skin with chlorhexidine; (3) Use maximal barrier precautions; (4) Avoid the femoral site; (5) Ask daily whether the benefits of the line exceed the risks.)
- *Implementation*: what is done to enable the units of change to adopt the change content (project group established, education, reminders, observation, performance feedback).

Is the intervention change itself complex or is the complexity in how we see it?

Enabling one physician to use a medication more selectively is usually a less complex endeavour than enabling all physicians in a health system to do so. Some changes are objectively more complex, when compared to other changes. But complexity also refers to how we perceive of a change: we can choose to understand a change in a more or less complex way. How we conceptualize a change is related to which data we collect and how we answer the evaluation customers' questions.

It is common in medical and health services research to understand a change as a cause, and to study effects using experimental research methods. This view of the intervention as a single cause of the outcomes is appropriate for answering a 'Does it make a difference?' question when all the other causes are controlled for.

But we can view the change as one of many influences affecting physicians, and operating in a system. This way of viewing is appropriate if we cannot control these other influences, and when answering other questions such as 'Will it work for us locally?' A 'systems view' expects this change to have delayed effects on physicians, and that physicians may take actions to modify the change itself. This is one of the different ways to conceptualize the change and its possible effects, each offering more or less complex ways of understanding the change.

This chapter regards 'complex social interventions' as changes which are objectively more complex, when compared to other changes. But also, that complexity resides in how we choose to view a change – we can understand it in a simple way, for example,as a cause and effect, or in a complex way, for example, as one influence in a dynamic system. No one way of viewing a change is better than another, but one way may be more useful in answering a specific question. Viewing a change as if it were a simple natural process, with the change as the cause and the outcome as an effect, may be useful for some purposes. Viewing it as a process subject to psychological, social and political processes may be useful for other purposes.

Challenges for describing and evaluating complex social interventions

Some evaluation challenges are unique to CSIs and some are more extreme versions of those faced by any evaluation. Below we note shortcomings described by previous research, and the challenges for evaluators.

Shortcomings of evaluations of CSIs

The first set of limitations described in the literature refers to an inadequate evaluation design for certainty about effects of the intervention. Many systematic reviews of evaluations of complex interventions assume the question is only, 'Did the CSI have an effect on important patient outcomes?', and assess an evaluation according to whether it used designs and methods thought to be best for identifying any such effects, such as an RCT. Thus Cochrane Reviews often note the limitations of many evaluations in relation to review criteria such as randomization, blinding, and control of confounders (EPOC 2009).

Practical: time, costs, randomization, controls and static standardization

Controlled trials take time and are costly to carry out. When the intervention is a change to provider units, randomization of these in sufficient numbers may be difficult to achieve. It may be difficult to agree beforehand on a set of controls not to receive the intervention. The intervention may be difficult to standardize or hold constant, and some interventions may need to be adapted during implementation in ways which cannot be pre-defined. Proponents of RCTs suggest that RCTs can accommodate being tailored to the situation, as in adjusting the dose to the patient, and have suggested different modifications to design which are described later.

In considering shortcomings, Kessler and Glasgow (2011) suggest about RCTs: 'when applied to the other major issues facing health care today, such trials are limited in their ability to address the complex populations and problems we face' and further state:

> A moratorium is proposed on such research for the next decade, and pragmatic, transparent, contextual, and multilevel designs that include replication, rapid learning systems and networks, mixed methods, and simulation and economic analyses to produce actionable, generalizable findings that can be implemented in real-world settings is suggested.

Descriptions: intervention and context is not described

One shortcoming noted by Campbell et al. (2000) is the lack of description about exactly what the intervention was and the setting in which it was implemented. This has also been noted in many other reviews (Michie et al. 2009).

Descriptions are needed to allow others to reproduce the CSI. One example is evaluations of dedicated stroke units, where there are often great variations in staff characteristics, clinical practices, management protocols and infrastructure. Another example is evaluations of rapid response teams, where there are similar variations. Without good descriptions of the intervention and the context, it is difficult to assess if the intervention was implemented fully, and as intended, or implemented in a context for which it was not designed.

This makes it difficult to judge generalizability: whether the intervention could be implemented elsewhere and if the results would be similar. Campbell et al.'s (2000) conclusions are not just regarding the need for better description, but also that 'unless the trials illuminate processes and mechanisms, they often fail to provide useful information'.

Outcomes: not explained by theory

One criticism is that many evaluations do not assess whether all the components of a CSI are needed or do not assess the contribution which each individually and together make to the outcomes. RCT designs in particular have been criticized for this, but a multi-arm randomized trial can be used to quantify the contributions of different components of a complex intervention (Altman 1991; Friedman and Wyatt 2006). Each arm of the trial exposes a group to an intervention component, or refers to the control group. If components of the intervention are not known, an expert panel can be used to define the potentially important components as a basis for the design (Friedman et al. 1998).

The above limitations found in descriptions are echoed in Glasziou et al. (2008) and in a review of 72 evaluations of quality improvement breakthrough programmes (Schouten et al. 2008). These involve project teams from different services meeting to learn and apply quality methods and to share experiences and results (Kilo 1998). This review first notes shortcomings arising from researchers not being able to apply adequate experimental design features, such as possible differences in baseline measurement between sites, limited data about the characteristics of control sites, no specification of blinded assessment, and possible contamination. But, in addition, Schouten et al. ask for more understanding of why there were variations of performance between the sites:

> The data collected in the included studies did not provide the information needed to understand and explain the findings. To understand how and why quality improvement collaboratives work, it is necessary to look into the 'black box' of the intervention and to study the determinants of success or failure.

Proponents of RCTs and many quasi-experimental designs argue that all you need to know is that it works, or that it works in a number of settings. This is countered by the argument that, for CSIs, as opposed to discrete prescribed interventions like medications, you may need to know why it works, and how it depends on or interacts with its environment, in order to reproduce it.

Common shortcomings of evaluations of complex social interventions

- *Implementation assessment failure*: The study does not examine the extent to which the programme was actually carried out. Was the intervention implemented fully, in all areas and to the required 'depth' and for how long?
- *Prestudy theory failure*: The study does not adequately review previous empirical or theoretical research to make explicit its theoretical framework, questions or hypotheses.
- *Outcome assessment failure*: The study does not assess a causal chain of outcomes or a sufficiently wide set of outcomes, such as short- and long-term impact on providers, organizations, patients, and resources, which would also detect unintended consequences.
- *Outcome attribution failure*: The study does not establish whether the outcomes can unambiguously be attributed to the intervention or list and assess other possible influences on outcomes.

- *Explanation theory failure*: There is no theory or model that explains how the intervention caused the outcomes and which factors and conditions were critical.
- *Measurement variability*: Different researchers use very different data to describe or measure the complex social intervention process, structure, and outcome. It is therefore difficult to use the results of one study to question or support another or to build up knowledge systematically (Øvretveit and Gustafson 2003).

Questions beyond 'does it work?' effectiveness questions

To be fair to recent discussions of experimental evaluations of complex interventions, they do emphasize the need for better descriptions, and also a better understanding of why there may be differences in outcomes between sites, and of the influences through which the intervention may have its effects (Glasgow et al. 2003; Glasziou et al. 2008; Fan et al. 2010; Schulz et al. 2010). The 'explanation criticism' made against experimental designs is unfair because experimental designs are not often designed to answer questions other than the 'does it work?' effectiveness question. However, wider discussions about making evaluations more relevant indicate the need to answer other questions beyond effectiveness: questions which practical implementers have, such as:

- What are the details of intervention and context?
- Do we have enough details to copy it and do we have the resources to do so? What are the details of both the content of the intervention change, and of the steps and actions to implement it, so that we could reproduce it in our setting?
- Are there controls in the study for ensuring implementation is carried out as described, and for excluding influences other than the intervention on the outcomes?
- Are there factors, apart from the intervention, which were helpful or necessary in order to carry out the intervention change, and which we need to know about to reproduce it in our setting?
- What was the role of researchers or others in assisting implementation and are additional specialists needed to reproduce the intervention in our setting?
- Are the methods to adapt the intervention to the setting described and reproducible in our setting, if adaptation is needed? Should we copy exactly the method for implementation rather than copy the content of the intervention?
- Is monitoring data on implementation and results necessary to adapt and check the intervention impact and, if so, which data, and can they be collected and reported easily and at low cost in our setting?
- How certain can we be of positive outcomes for our patients if the outcomes are process of care outcomes which are 'thought to ensure improved patient outcomes'?
- If we did copy it, could we expect similar outcomes or are there context influences that would affect the outcomes in our setting?

- Have the costs to implement, operate and maintain the intervention change been estimated, and is it economically feasible for us?
- Can we reproduce the resources and necessary conditions for implementation and sustainability in our setting?

Challenges for experimental evaluations of complex interventions

Experimental evaluations focus on answering the 'Is it effective?' question. Usually these designs concentrate on a few measures of effectiveness and collect these data 'before' and 'after' the intervention to assess if the intervention has made a difference to these measures. The designs use different methods to assess how certain we can be that difference between the 'before' and 'after' data are caused by the intervention rather than by something else. These designs include the randomized controlled trial design, matched comparison trials, pragmatic trials, 'before' and 'after' evaluations with no comparisons, and other designs (MRC 2000; Tunis et al. 2003; Mercer et al. 2007; Craig et al. 2008; Fan et al. 2010).

Researchers using these designs to answer the 'is it effective?' question face the following challenges, which are not unique to complex interventions but may arise in a more extreme form

- *Describing the intervention and the different components*, including how much of the implementation actions to include in the definition of the intervention.

  For example, for an intervention to an ICU to prevent central line blood stream infections (CLABSI), is the intervention only the changes to clinical practice, or does it also include changes previously made to the ICU which make it easier consistently to follow the new clinical practice, such as a clinical unit safety programme (Pronovost et al. 2008; AHRQ 2011)?

  A description is needed for others to understand what the intervention was and to reproduce it if they choose to. Trials of simple clinical interventions have also been criticized for not giving sufficient descriptions (Begg et al. 1996; Schulz et al. 2010).

  If it is essential for implementers to adapt an intervention it in an undefined way, how to document the adaptation? Physicians adjust doses according to trial protocol, but implementers have far less precise guidance and greater latitude in how to adapt some CSIs.
- *Deciding which outcomes* would indicate effectiveness, and how to capture any indications of unexpected and unwanted outcomes:

  Which possible effects of a CLABSI intervention to an ICU can be measured or documented, and which are most relevant to the evaluation user's decisions? Is there evidence that intermediate or process data, such as orders for medications for treating blood stream infections, are reliable and valid indicators of the effects of the intervention? Should the evaluation collect data about costs and possible savings? If the intervention is at multiple levels, which outcome data should be collected? Should data on many outcomes be collected or should researcher resources be concentrated on collecting fewer outcomes with more validity and reliability?

The 'causal chain' from intervention to patient or cost outcomes may be through a number of intermediate stages. This requires that outcomes are collected at each stage of the causal chain to trace final impact (Nazareth et al. 2002). Or can the evaluation rely only on evidence from other research that achieving an intermediate outcome is predictive of likely impact on later outcomes?

- *Randomization* of subjects to receive the intervention and its comparison may be difficult when these are individual providers, service teams or units or health systems.

  If the number of possible providers or units is small (e.g. 30 or fewer), randomization does not distribute sufficient numbers to 'experimental' and 'control' groups to allow sufficient certainty about whether outcome differences between the groups are due to the intervention or something else.
- Alternatively, *matching* intervention and comparison groups to reduce confounding influences also may be difficult. This is especially so if there is no evidence or theory about which characteristics of providers or services may make them more or less susceptible to influence by the intervention.

Generally, an evaluation study or an evaluation design can only answer one or a few questions, and its validity is judged in terms of how well it answers these questions. A randomized controlled trial (RCT) is often the best design for answering the question, 'What were the effects of this intervention on the recipient in terms of these measured variables . . .?' It is the worst design for answering questions such as, 'How did the intervention evolve over time and which factors influenced this evolution?' Thus, the shortcomings of an evaluation are in relation to the question it set out to answer.

Challenges for evaluations of complex social interventions

Critics of the experimental approach to evaluation have proposed that, in addition to the challenges noted above, there are further challenges which arise because the 'social' nature of the intervention is such a central part of it (Greenhalgh et al. 2004; Ferlie et al. 2005; Dixon-Woods et al. 2011; Øvretveit 2011a). These criticisms arise from these authors way of conceptualizing CSIs as:

- a series of actions carried out by human beings, with varying intensity and quality;
- influences on other human beings, who have choice, and are exposed to competing influences;
- features in a changing social, economic and political situation which affects people's actions and responses.

The actions of a pharmaceutical or surgical treatment can be described as a 'mechanism' which operates according to natural laws of physiology, which are largely independent of what a person thinks about it. Actions such as education, feedback, financial incentives, or directives depend for their effects on how individuals interpret the meaning of the action. A directive to nurses to wear a sign saying 'Do not interrupt while preparing and dispensing medications' was not worn by some nurses, who interpreted this as an insult to their intelligence, and another action by management to be resisted because it showed disrespect to their professionalism.

There is a regularity in how people, groups and organizations interpret the intervention actions to influence them, and in the outcomes of the intervention because individuals share group norms and cultures. However, the outcomes are still less predictable than those from a mechanical or physiological action on a human body. In addition, the social world of which the individuals and groups are part of changes in a way in which the human body does not, and in ways which are significant for how the implementation actions are interpreted. A series of articles in a nursing journal about 'Do not interrupt' signs, and a recommendation by a safety association persuaded more nurses that this was good nursing practice and not an insult to their intelligence and professionalism.

There are often many outcomes which are of interest to one evaluation user group or to different stakeholders. Often qualitative data about outcomes is the only feasible data collection strategy, such as documenting informed observers' assessments of whether the outcome was achieved and the evidence they give for their assessments.

Complex social interventions often comprise a series of actions, as, for example, in a health promotion campaign for a 'healthy lifestyle' (e.g. HealthyPeople.gov 2011). The desired effects depend on the intervention actions being carried out, as well as the social conditions which support the actions: the degree to which the actions can be fully and consistently carried out depends on the conditions surrounding the actors, such as higher-level support, resources, time, knowledge and skills. The effects of these actions also depend on conditions which help or hinder the actions to have the desired results (e.g. media or cultural influences which contradict or complement the actions and which interact with the actions). The sustainability of such interventions and their results depend even more on the surrounding conditions – short-term evaluations are less sensitive to the role of surrounding conditions and how they change. To understand which conditions are necessary for implementation and desired effects, it does not always help to 'control these out' as 'confounders'. It may be better to understand how they have their influence.

As a result of these considerations, some evaluation researchers seek to answer questions other than the, 'Is it effective?' question, and use methods which seek to understand how the intervention 'causes' its effects. These methods give more recognition to the social nature of the intervention.

This alternative way to conceptualize CSIs leads some evaluators who hold these ideas to be reluctant to use the term 'intervention', which to them suggests a discrete, isolatable force, aimed at 'targets', viewed as objects in their response. Instead subjects are viewed as 'taking up' the 'intervention' resources or ideas offered, if they choose to do so, and creatively applying it in their setting. 'Intervention' is regarded more as 'facilitated uptake' by active subjects who may then make innovations to the intervention which can make it more or less effective than it would otherwise be in their setting. Indeed, 'evaluation' is viewed by some using this idea as a less useful term than 'enabling continuous learning for improvement'.

A summary of CSI challenges

Some CSIs can be prescribed, implemented with fidelity to the prescription and evaluated using experimental designs and controls. However, such designs may not be appropriate for other CSIs, and for other questions because:

- Replication of a complex intervention may be more difficult elsewhere: requirements for standardization and control needed in the study design may be difficult to achieve in routine practice.
- Prescription of the intervention components may not be appropriate. Implementation often require implementers to revise the intervention in ways which cannot be prescribed, but guidance can be given for methods for making adaptations. Description of the changes and methods used in practice is thus necessary, which may call for refocusing the evaluation on other outcomes than those originally planned.
- The time taken for the study may be too long for practice and policy, especially for evaluations of changes which involve rapidly-developing technologies.
- To inform their actions, stakeholders have a need for information in addition to 'Is the intervention effective for producing these selected outcomes?'
- For these and other reasons, observational and action evaluation designs are needed, but these have their shortcomings and are not as well understood as experimental designs.

Choices for research design for evaluating CSIs

Other chapters of the book have described experimental, observational and action-oriented evaluation designs. This section considers in more detail the theory-informed observational or action-oriented approaches for evaluating CSIs, which provide more understanding of the social aspects of these interventions, and may provide some answers to the questions noted above which experimental evaluations were unable to answer.

Frameworks, models and theory in evaluating CSIs

It is becoming good practice for most types of CSI evaluation to use a model, theory or framework to guide the study. These help to define which data to collect and can be used to develop explanations for how or why the intervention has the effects discovered in different settings. Such explanations can help users to apply or adapt the intervention to their setting or to judge if they are likely to be able to implement it at all.

These models are theories or assumptions about the actions and conditions needed to produce certain outcomes. They are diagrams of either the intervention or of the main parts of the evaluation. The theory may be those of the evaluators, as they try to conceptualize or map the intervention, its context, and their expectations of outcomes. Or it may be the assumptions of the implementers or designers, which the evaluators discover by interviewing them or by studying plans. Or it may be a combination of the evaluator's and the implementer's ideas.

Different terms are used, but here we refer to the two types of model in this way: the programme theory (or logic model) and the evaluation model (or framework).

The programme theory or logic model

Figure 12.1 shows the most important ingredients which are thought to be needed to carry out the intervention and the intermediate and later outcomes expected. Sometimes this is referred to as the 'model' or 'framework' for the intervention.

This can serve as a framework which maps which types of data to collect, so as to assess whether the items which are assumed to be needed for the outcomes were implemented. Then as an aid to decide which outcomes to study.

A programme theory or logic model helps map which types of data to collect, so as to assess whether the items that are assumed to be needed for the outcomes have been implemented. The framework can then be used to decide which outcomes to study.

The evaluation model or framework

Figure 12.2 is a diagram of the evaluation which shows the items on which data will be collected, which are needed to describe and assess the outcomes of the intervention. The design diagram sometimes serves as an evaluation model or framework.

There are three key points to note:

- The implementation or evaluation models show: the intervention (its component parts, or which activities are undertaken), the expected outcomes, and sometimes the context of the intervention.

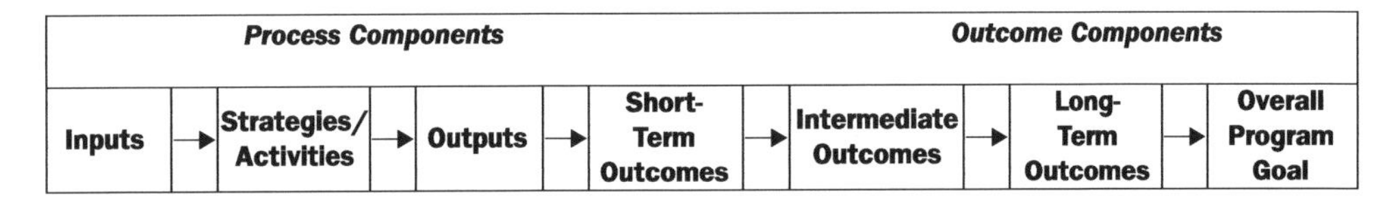

Figure 12.1 The programme theory or logic model

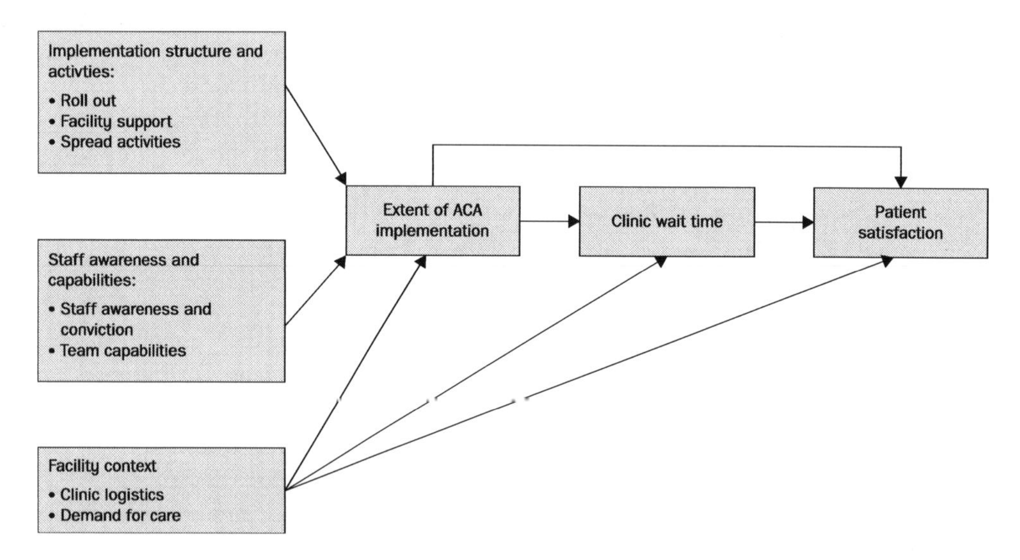

Figure 12.2 The implementation and effectiveness of advanced clinic access: evaluation model
Source: Van Deusen Lukas et al. (2004).

- The boxes summarize ideas about the activities and ingredients which are expected to produce different outcomes. This then lays the basis for the evaluator to specify further which data or measures need to be collected to assess if these were implemented or present, and the methods and times for data collection.
- One way in which the models differ is in the extent to which they list 'context factors' which may be needed for the intervention to be implemented.

What about context?

The first example with the logic model above (CDC 2008) does not have a box describing the 'context' of the intervention. This may be because the proposers of the model do not think context will have any influence over whether the intervention can be implemented. It may be because the users are only interested in the effectiveness in one setting.

However, research shows that many CSIs have different outcomes in different settings, primarily because the setting affects how much of the intervention is implemented. Understanding which context factors helped and hindered implementation allows the evaluator to give some guidance about the settings in which the intervention can be implemented, and about where and when similar results could be expected – it enables an assessment of generalizability.

The second model – the evaluation model (Van Deusen Lukas et al. 2004) – has a box describing 'facility context', which includes 'clinic logistics' and 'demand for care'. These are two things the evaluators want to examine to find out how much these affect implementation, as well as clinic wait times and patient satisfaction. These context factors are not the intervention (which is 'advanced clinic access'), but they are thought to affect its implementation and the outcomes.

The model also has two other 'context' boxes for 'staff awareness and capabilities' and 'implementation structure and activities'. The evaluators theorize that these affect the extent to which the advance clinic access intervention will be implemented.

Further details of the evaluation show which data were collected to document and quantify these context factors, as well as document the intervention implemented and its outcomes.

More detailed context frameworks

There are more detailed and sophisticated models and frameworks on the aspects of context which are thought to influence the implementation of different classes of complex social intervention. These can give a starting point for evaluators to decide which aspects of a context to study and which data and measures to use to collect data about these aspects.

For interventions of evidence-based clinical changes, a well-developed framework of different elements of context is given in the PARiHS model (Stetler et al. 2011).

'Readiness for change' is one aspect of context which can be measured and which can help evaluations of CSIs in natural settings to explain findings and to give guidance to users. Again, which factors to examine depends on the type of CSI being evaluated. Different factors may be important in implementing a computer decision support system from those for implementing a resident fall prevention programme in a nursing home. A general framework and measure for collecting data about readiness for change are found in the ORCA instrument (Helfrich et al. 2009).

As regards context for quality improvement CSIs in primary care (which includes a wide range of interventions), Brennan et al.'s (2012) review provides one model and a more detailed list of context factors (51 measurement instruments). Another framework which can serve as a starting point for the evaluation of some quality improvement or similar CSIs is the Model for Understanding Success in Quality (MUSIQ) (Kaplan et al. 2011). These are summarized in Øvretveit (2013).

Issues to consider in applying designs to evaluate CSIs

The chapter has considered some of the shortcomings of previous evaluations of CSIs in answering different questions. In recent years the field has developed a greater understanding of the range of questions which evaluations of CSI sometimes need to address, and that some designs can never satisfactorily answer certain questions. This summary notes some of the issues to consider raised by different commentaries and studies and is based on the principles for user-centred evaluation described in Part I of the book.

Define the information needed by users of the evaluation

As with most evaluations, the starting point is to identify the information needed and formulate a question in a way which can be answered adequately by any evaluation design, given the constraints. If the evaluation is to focus on providing practical actors with information to make decisions about the CSI, then the evaluators and the users together need to list what information would be needed to better inform decisions where the evaluation could help. The evaluator's role may include helping users to list the information needed and consider whether this information would make a difference for practical decisions and actions. The evaluator has in mind different designs and the costs and time-delivery parameters of these designs, and can show the users what is possible by when and for how much. The process leads to agreement on information to be collected by the evaluation, the questions it will answer and its purpose.

The two aims of answering practical questions in a timely and actionable way and contributing to scientific knowledge can be achieved by one evaluation design. But it is challenging to do so, and it may be that the evaluator has to focus on achieving only one of these aims.

Choose the design to answer the questions and provide the information

Whether the question is primarily practice-action driven or research-science driven, the choice of design should follow from the question. Evaluators tend to specialize in particular methods and designs and may be blind to the possibility that another design is more suited to the question. The much-needed innovation in designs for evaluating CSIs to answer a range of questions requires all evaluators to consider modifications or hybrid designs which they may not have used before.

Understand and describe the limitations to the design for answering some questions

This is necessary to avoid others being misled by the evaluation findings in the final report. But, at the start, defining the limitations can help innovation in design and method by sensitizing evaluators to possible data or strategies that could help the evaluation and provide answers to questions which it may not have otherwise been able to answer.

Recognize and address challenges which readers may have in using the evaluation

The point about researchers being unfamiliar with some designs and methods also applies to readers. Evaluations published in specialist journals can often assume the average reader of such journals is able to understand the design and judge the significance and applicability of the results. Evaluation reports for a wider academic readership, or primarily for non-researchers, need to provide discussion of the design and methods which is not only more detailed but is also simplified and understandable for readers with a knowledge of other designs, or of none at all.

In some cases, the evaluator might not use a design if the user may not be able to understand and apply the findings generated by it, or because the evaluator honestly recognizes that they cannot present the design in a usable way. This applies equally to some quantitative analytic methods as to long narratives from qualitative or realist evaluations, which in theory are well suited to CSI evaluation but are difficult for some researchers to communicate or summarize.

Pay attention to each of the 'ADAGU' questions

Overall, it is best when designing the evaluation to note the strategies which can and will be used within the evaluation to address each of these questions below. Stating these strategies will strengthen proposals for funditng the evaluation, help in developing innovations in design, and make the final report more useful:

- Aims: what information is needed and what are the questions to be addressed?
- Description: what are the details of intervention, implementation and context?
- Attribution: how certain can we be that the intervention caused the outcomes reported?
- Generalization: can we copy it and get similar results?
- Usefulness: in which situations can it be used?

Conclusion

It may be necessary to consider the social aspect of complex interventions in order better to answer evaluation users' questions. There is authoritative guidance on evaluating complex interventions but these have their shortcomings with regard to understanding the social aspects of the intervention, and in producing actionable knowledge. The chapter showed that many interventions to healthcare, to patients and to populations are not only complex but social interventions: the 'social' emphasizes specific dynamics and an unpredictability which need to be considered by evaluators. The cost and time increasingly invested in CSIs demand more resources be allocated to their evaluation. The chapter calls for improving evaluation methods and evaluator skills to answer different evaluation questions so as to help users make more informed decisions about whether and how to implement an intervention.

Awareness of the range of designs, and of better ways to formulate answerable evaluation questions, makes it more likely evaluators will better match design to the purpose of and constraints on the evaluation. Other developments are needed, such as more attention to formulating questions and goals for the evaluation, formulating programme theory before data-gathering, and attention to context, reporting standards and costing.

13 Evaluating return on investment and value improvements

Introduction

Is a change worth the cost and effort it takes to make the change? This depends on your perspective, and what you value. This chapter considers how to evaluate the return on investment (ROI) of a change: whether a change 'pays back', for whom, and when. It also considers how to evaluate whether something is a 'value improvement', that is, whether it both improves quality and uses fewer resources.

The evaluation designs described in the chapter can be used for a pre-appraisal, to help decide before making a change whether the likely savings or gains are worth the costs. Pre-appraisals also help to specify what is to be expected and the monitoring data so that, if the change is made, then it can be managed more effectively to produce a return on the investment.

The designs can also be retrospective, to look back and evaluate the returns produced by an investment in a change, and to decide whether to invest in future similar changes. They can also be used prospectively, to plan an evaluation of the costs and returns of a proposed change. The knowledge can then be used in various ways, including re-adjusting the share of the financial costs and gains between different parties involve in the change.

In the past, few health and healthcare evaluations have considered ROI. Resource issue, such as the cost of a change or the value of the results, have usually been assessed using academic health economic evaluation methods (Drummond et al. 1987). ROI estimations are a simple type of cost-benefit evaluation, limited to considering only the resources spent and saved by the investor, which is often a provider, a health system or another financing body. They are one type of cost benefit analysis.

In theory, the 'investment' could be any human or natural resource used for the intervention, and which could be used for other purposes. The 'return' could be any benefit which has value such as the time saved for a family member of a patient, or less use of a scarce natural resource. This chapter describes first the most limited ROI evaluations, which take a provider or health system investor perspective. These consider the largest and most easily quantifiable resources invested (often personnel time) and focus on those which can be expressed in money terms. They consider the results of the change or intervention which the resources are given for, and focus on those which can be expressed in money terms and realized as 'cash pay-back' for the investment.

The chapter then considers a broader type of ROI evaluation which considers both the quality and the resource returns of an investment, so as to evaluate whether an intervention is a 'value improvement'.

An example of an ROI

'What is the return on investment for starting a nurse case management service for children with asthma who have a high risk of serious, but avoidable, asthma attacks?' This was a question asked in a study of projects for certain patient populations in 10 US Medicaid-managed care organizations (Greene et al. 2008). The study found that the investment costs for this programme were US$126,151. The savings after three years were US$801,345, giving a three-year ROI of over 1:6.

The three-year ROI in the example of 1:6 means that for every US$1 invested in this programme, the ROI evaluation estimated it would save the managed care organization US$6 over a three-year period. This was because the cost of the nurse case management service was six times less costly than the emergency room and hospital admissions which would otherwise have occurred over three years – as indicated by the comparison patients and services without this service.

To answer the question, the example had to specify whose perspective (the managed care organization), and which time period was considered (three years). These are two important considerations in return on investment evaluations because the investments and returns or benefits are different if you are a provider, or purchaser or another party. The return on investment is different one year after the start of the investment to the return after three years: first, it can take up to 12 months to establish the change as fully operational; second, the start-up costs which make most of the investment are in the early stages, and the returns, if there are any, are only beginning. After three years the start-up investment costs have disappeared, leaving the running costs as the only investment cost.

The difference between theoretical and cash savings

A third point to note is the difference between 'theoretical' costs and savings and the 'end-of-year budget' costs and savings. This research did not collect financial data from different operating units' budgets to find out exactly how much each unit had spent and saved. Thus, it neither estimated the impact on operating units' budgets, nor did it collect data about exactly what this impact was.

Actual savings can be very different to theoretical savings. Those making estimations typically do not consider all the extra changes which may be needed to redeploy staff or close beds in order to realize end-of-year budget savings, and these changes are often difficult and costly. Saved time and materials have to be turned into cash. Time-based budget impact analysis (BIA) techniques can be used to make these estimations and can be used to track actual impacts at different points in the year. The principles of BIA are used in the evaluation steps in the ROI guidance given next.

How to carry out a simple return on investment evaluation

The evaluation can be carried out retrospectively, if the evaluator can find sufficiently detailed and valid information from historical records and databases.

Ideally, the evaluation is planned and prospective, which makes it possible to identify the data needed beforehand and set up systems to gather or extract the data.

1 *Define the change* which the investments will be used to make. In the example, this is a nurse case management service for children with asthma with a high risk of serious, avoidable asthma attacks.
2 *List the time and other resources needed* (a) to make the change; and (b) to sustain the change once it is made. First, to establish this nurse case management service, a project team is needed to plan the service, set up the systems for running the service, recruit nurses and to make it operational. Second, when it becomes operational, the service will have a cost to run, involving staff salaries, and the costs of maintaining and running the systems.
3 *Define the investment and the investor.* Decide how much time and how many resources the investor is to contribute and quantify the money value of these. These are the costs which the investor will pay, of the costs of what needs to be added to establish and sustain the intervention. In the example, the investor will be taken to be a managed care organization (typically a health system of a hospital, primary care providers and other services). In the study cited, the investors were actually (a) a separate research funding agency which provided most of the funding to establish and evaluate the system; and (b) the managed care organization which contributed some of the resources to set up the care management system.
4 *Define the returns to be valued.* Identify the benefits important to the investor, usually those which provide cash returns to the investor. In the example, these are any savings or extra costs to the health system investing in the care management service. A managed care organization is paid a set fee per member and so the organization has to bear the costs of most services and sometimes of medications needed by any member. The returns to be valued are the savings which result from less use of services. These are indicated by previous research into similar case management services. These are PCP, emergency room, hospital inpatient and outpatient services, medications and any other services provided by the health system which could be affected by the care management service.
5 *Decide the ROI study design and data.* This involves defining the methods to assess whether the 'returns' were primarily due to the investment change and not due to some other influence. Then, it involves deciding which data to gather, from which sources using which methods and when, to find out: (a) how many of the resources the investor paid for were invested, of those resources defined earlier in point (3); (b) how many returns were realized and when those resources were as defined earlier in point (4). In the example, the design was a comparative before/after study with patients receiving case management matched to patients who did not receive this service. It is possible to use a before/after design without comparison, but there will be less certainty that the result returns are due to the investment-intervention. The data gathered about the investment were data on:

   The costs of the project to set up the case management service, gathered by interviewing project team members and assigning salary and other costs of the project and new systems needed.

The annual operating costs of the new service, which involved listing the main elements and assigning costs to these.

The data gathered about the 'returns' were data on services used by case management and non-case management controls: one year of baseline 'before' data and two years of post-intervention billing data were used for hospital care, physician services in all settings, home care, long-term care, hospital ER use, and prescription drugs.

6 *Collect and analyse the data and present*: (a) investment costs and time period of investment; (b) returns at year 1 from start of investment, and at years 2 and 3; (c) ROI at three years. In the example the investment costs for this programme were US$126,151. This was the cost to set up, and then run the programme for three years (annual operating costs were cumulatively added). The savings over three years were US$801,345, in fewer services and medications than the control patients. The three-year ROI was thus at least 1:6.
7 *Specify assumptions, limits and degree of certainty of the evaluation.* This means stating assumptions are made about (a) factors other than the investment change which may contribute to result returns; (b) data validity – mostly costing data. From this statement of assumptions, the evaluator can say how confident they are about the upper and lower limits of their estimates. In the case example, the statement may be 'investment and savings could vary by + or –12%; and the ROI at three years could be between 1:5 and 1:7. NIII (2011) gives details and examples of sources of data in the UK NHS as well as a guide ROI calculator.

Is a 'return on investment' evaluation the same as a 'business case' assessment?

An ROI evaluation is part of many business case assessments. A business case also involves other statements about why the investment comes within the mission of an organization, and why it contributes to strategic objectives or to other changes being made at the same time. A business case is where the justification, plan and expected results are laid out in one document. It might include statements about:

- current problems and opportunities;
- a change and how and why it will solve the problem facing the organization and contribute to strategic objectives;
- the time, money and other resources needed from the organization and from others to make the change successfully;
- expected benefits especially in relation to the current problem or strategy, and expected ROI at one, three, and five years;
- risks and risk management strategies;
- the expected situation if the change is not undertaken, and the possible alternative use of the resources proposed for the change;
- an outline draft plan for next steps.

Reiter et al. (2007) give a more detailed summary of how to formulate a business case for a quality improvement or similar change.

Evaluating value improvements

Value improvements are changes which both improve quality and reduce waste, and usually reduce the costs of producing a service. Evaluations are needed to assess whether promising changes do in fact improve quality and reduce waste. They are also needed to assess whether the cost of the change is worth the improved quality and reduced waste which the change may produce. Evaluations of value improvements thus assess the costs of a supposed improvement and the quality results and resource results.

One type of evaluation of a value improvement is a 'Cost-Quality Return on Investment' evaluation (CQROI) (Øvretveit 2012). It is more limited than a full cost-effectiveness or cost-utility health economics research study. But it is broader than the ROI evaluation described above because it considers both the quality returns and the resource returns. Return on investment evaluations usually only consider the pay-back for the investor in terms of the money they get back for the money they put in, at a certain 'pay-back date'.

Evaluating cost-quality return on investment for promising value improvement

An example of a 'value improvement' is a hospital providing information to primary care about the patients' medication and after-care details to the primary care provider (PCP). Previous research has found this can improve quality and may reduce costs. This change can avoid suffering for the patient because it makes it less likely that a PCP will give the wrong after-care or medications, and can also avoid unnecessary readmission or visits to the primary care provider. From the patient's perspective and from the payer's perspective, it improves the quality of care and reduces waste and costs for them. Note, though, that under some payment systems it results in lost income for the providers: many systems will pay the hospital and PCP for the extra work which could have been avoided by this improved patient discharge system. Thus, who makes or loses money from a value improvement depends on the financing system, who makes the investment and how long is the time period considered.

Box 13.1 An example evaluating value improvements: operation cancellations and delays in a Norwegian hospital (Øvretveit 2000)

If a patient has been prepared for an operation, either psychologically or biophysically, for example, with antibiotic prophylaxis, then a delay or cancellation can be frustrating, at best. It can also be costly:

1 'Cost of the problem' to the hospital: 98 cancellations every three months resulting on average of 20 minutes' wasted time for the operating room team = a cost of US$320,000 annually.

2 'Spend cost': in the first year of a quality project was US$98,000 which was the cost of members' time in a project team and the

cost to set up a simple system to record and feed-back delays and cancellations.

3 'Savings' in staff time resulting from a 20 per cent reduction in cancellations was US$64,000. The ROI evaluation found that these time savings could be used to treat more patients, bringing a consequent increase in hospital income. A rough estimation was that the increased income from the time released was US$92,000 each year.

4 The ROI for the first year was negative or a loss, because the spend cost that year of US$98,000 was not paid back by the time saved and the extra patients treated. It was only by month 7 that the changes that the team had made began to result in a drop in cancellation rates. However, it took time to increase the number of patients treated so that the save time could be turned into increased cash income.

5 The three-year ROI was positive because the spend cost of US$98,000 was paid back during the second year. This was because there were no project team costs or ongoing costs to sustain the 20 per cent reduction in cancellations. And the saved time could be fully converted into treating extra patients (the time savings were 'monetized'). By year 3, the increased income was US$92,000 and continued into subsequent years compared to the start of year 1.

The evaluation found that the intervention was a value improvement, giving a QCROI payback after ten months of the investment, and providing a monetized value improvement for the ICU and hospital budgets by year 2.

Box 13.2 Predicting value improvement

The third evaluation method described here is a way of assessing from previous research or information whether a change will be a value improvement. The method used in Øvretveit (2012) and Øvretveit (2013) to make 'value improvement estimates' was as follows:

Problems: waste and costs

1 For studies with evidence of problems, select those which quantify the problems or a problem. Use these to estimate the possible waste or cost to providers or health systems, showing the basis for the estimate and the limitations. Emphasize that the figure is

an estimation by giving a range estimate (i.e. 'unlikely that this would cost a provider less than . . . or more than . . .').

Solutions: their cost, and likely savings (or loss)

2 For intervention studies, exclude those interventions and studies with inadequate evidence of quality improvements (i.e. the evidence is not sufficiently strong, or there is strong evidence of no improvement, for intermediate or final outcomes such as patient experience/satisfaction or effective care practices/process and clinical outcomes).

3 Identify studies with acceptable evidence of quality improvement and also some evidence of resources or cost, and include and summarize these in the review.

4 For studies with evidence of quality improvements only, identify whether they provide any data to allow some estimate of resources used for the intervention, and or resources saved (e.g. number of emergency department visits, physician office visits, hospital days or length of stay, medications supplied, other consumable or equipment costs). Then make an estimate of the extra time saved or spent.

Value improvement estimation for local services

The following summarizes a method which a local service can use to make a prediction of whether a reported change would result in a value improvement in the service (Øvretveit 2012):

1 Does previous research or information give 'strong enough' evidence of quality improvement? If yes, then, continue with points 2–7.
2 How much does the intervention cost (investment)?
3 Is there any evidence of reductions in waste and more efficient use of resources (e.g. fewer visits/admissions, fewer medications/tests, shorter length of stay, time saved)?
4 What is the money value of these reductions and efficiencies?
5 If there is no evidence from research for points 2, or 3, then use theory or estimations for deciding a cost range (e.g. it is likely that the spend cost would not be less than £X and not more than £X).
6 Overall, what is the return on investment, if any, for a particular stakeholder (The stakeholder ROI means: what is the cost of the change and savings or extra cost for different stakeholders (patient, providers, payer, or integrated health system)?)

7 Time to pay off: How are the spendings and savings distributed between different parties at year 1, year 2, year 3, year 5 or year 10?

Summary: key points

Remember, a 'good' ROI evaluation does the following:

- Specifies the user of the evaluation and the decisions the evaluation will inform.
- Identifies all the costs and benefits which are important to the users' decisions, and measures in financial terms those which are feasible to measure.
- Distinguishes in the findings the theoretical ROI and also the actual or likely monetized ROI (based on actual cash savings) at different times after the intervention starts.
- Specifies the limitations, assumptions and range of certainty of the results.

Conclusion

The chapter has shown how to carry out a simple financial return on investment evaluation for an intervention or a change. This can be used as part of a business case or to help decide data to collect and what to expect when managing implementation. It also showed how to make a value improvement evaluation to assess the return on investment of a change which is intended to raise quality and reduce waste. The third method described was one which can be used when considering research or reports about improvements, and to predict likely ROI from the available data. The concepts and definitions are listed in the Glossary.

For most interventions or changes, the ROI changes over time. This is because, initially, is an investment to plan and make the change. Over time this start-up 'spend cost' becomes less, but there will then be the routine recurring cost of operating and sustaining the change. For a change to give a return on investment, the cost of both making and sustaining the change must be paid for by the savings or extra income from the changed situation, and this often takes till the second or third year to achieve with even the better ROI changes. As regards savings or extra income, this will depend on whether the time or materials savings identified can be turned into cash – typically by treating more patients or closing beds.

14 Economic evaluation

Introduction

Economic evaluations are often combined with, or built onto experimental evaluations. Some understanding of the principles of economic evaluation is important even for those who will never carry out or use an economic evaluation. Most health evaluations need to pay attention to the resources used by, and the consequences of, an intervention. Many economic concepts and ways of thinking are helpful in designing an evaluation study and also in deciding how to act on the findings.

Are they unethical? A surprising question, but economic evaluations can raise strong passions. There are those who argue that not to look at the costs of an intervention is irresponsible because it ignores how the money could be spent on other things. Yet there are those who oppose 'reducing everything to money' – that different interventions cannot be compared or valued in 'simplistic' terms, and doing so hides the assumptions of the calculations behind apparently objective and precise figures. And, it is true that, after following the relentless logic from calculating the costs of nurses' time through to the value of a year of life expressed as a number, we seem to have missed something along the way – it all makes perfect sense, but it feels senseless. But, with some medications now costing US$100,000 – for one year – we need to ask, what are the benefits compared to this cost, and what resources might that take away from other uses? Similarly, for health reforms – do we even know what they cost?

Economic evaluations can make it easier for people to avoid the painful and complex work of weighing up the many considerations in judging the value of an intervention. But they can also give information about the use of resources and this is essential for making judgements of value. We as health workers and as citizens increasingly need to confront the unthinking choices which we do make, and would rather not make consciously.

This chapter will not equip you to carry out an economic evaluation, but it will introduce you to the concepts and principles of the economic perspective, and to the main types of economic evaluation study: cost description, cost minimization, cost consequence description, cost-effectiveness, cost utility and finally cost-benefit – the last being a term which is incorrectly used to describe almost any economic analysis. The chapter will also sensitize you to the assumptions underlying different types of study, because there is virtually no one working in the health sector – and increasingly patients as well – who do not now need to be able to assess the strengths and weaknesses of an economic evaluation.

The economic perspective

Economists are philosophers of scarcity. The economic perspective focuses on how many resources are used by an intervention and on the consequences of the intervention which can be quantified. Yet to define the economic perspective only in this way is to omit the most important assumption of the perspective, which is that the resources used by an intervention could always be put to other uses, or rather that the resources are being withheld from other uses. This is the concept of 'opportunity cost', which lies at the heart of the economic perspective, and which forces us to recognize choices.

A more accurate definition of economic evaluation is 'the comparative analysis of alternative courses of action in terms of both the costs and consequences', where the alternative could even be no action (Drummond et al. 1987). The consequences include the effects on a patient or on the beneficiary of the intervention. Sometimes 'consequences' include resources which are saved or used as a result of the intervention by patients (e.g. travel costs), their families, a health service and society.

Economic evaluations differ in the ways in which they assess costs and consequences and in what they include and exclude in their costing and consequences assessments (the 'scope' of the evaluation). Figure 14.1 uses a time-line to show the different types of economic evaluation underneath the aspect of the intervention's inputs, outputs and outcomes which is the focus of the evaluation.

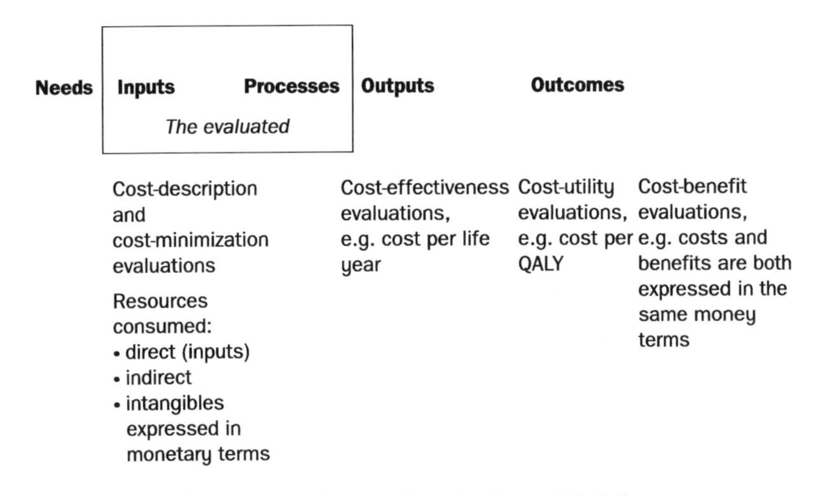

Figure 14.1 Different types of economic evaluation and their focus

Cost-description and cost-minimization evaluations

Cost-minimization evaluations are limited cost descriptions. These descriptions and cost minimization evaluations only calculate the resources used in interventions ('inputs'), and usually quantify these resources in money terms. This makes it easier to compare the total resources used by different interventions.

Examples are cost-description evaluations of inpatient care compared to day care. In an old, but still interesting study, Marks et al. (1980) report retrospective costing of a range of procedures, including 'breast biopsy and partial mastectomy', finding that inpatient costs for the latter were on average $210, compared to 'day patient' costs of $26.

Note that many cost evaluations only describe the costs of one intervention, and are thus termed 'partial' evaluations because they do not explicitly compare the intervention with one or more alternatives. In economic evaluations, 'description' usually means description of one intervention and not a comparison: for example, a cost description of the resources consumed by a new drug treatment for asthma, or a nursing service, or a new personnel overtime policy. A 'cost-consequence description' is also a 'partial' economic evaluation because, though it considers consequences as well as costs, it does not compare the intervention with alternatives. However, there is an implicit comparison because the costs of the one intervention are expressed in money terms, and this invites comparisons with other uses of the money, though many of these other uses may not have been so precisely costed.

Cost description is similar to what many of us do when we calculate the costs of a proposed or past action. But it involves two things which we do not usually do when looking at the cost of, for example, a holiday. First, a cost description calculates accurately the cost of all resources consumed by the health service, for example, the cost of all staff time and materials, electricity, administration and other 'overheads'. Second, it often lists a range of other costs, such as to other welfare services, to patients and relatives and to society, as well as the 'intangible costs'. The resources used which are described depend on the perspective of the study: the three most common are the health service, the patient and the societal perspective. It is the duty of the evaluator to draw attention to the perspective taken and to note the resources used which are important to other perspectives.

We note that this simplest of economic evaluations makes many assumptions about how to quantify the resources consumed by one intervention, and, if two or more are compared, how to equate and compare the resources consumed. There are assumptions about what to include in the cost of 'overheads' (is training included?) and in the costs of capital and rate of depreciation. There are questions about how broad the scope of the costing should be: should it include environmental costs?

Economists have different views about which costs should be considered as direct, indirect and intangible, and about the breadth of scope of costing. A technique called 'sensitivity analysis' is useful because it allows us to vary an assumption to see how it affects the results of the study, for example, a graph which shows how varying the costs charged for 'overheads' affects the total cost of an intervention. However, we should really call calculating costs 'economic valuation', so that we remind ourselves that it is not a technical value-free procedure, but involves many assumptions.

Cost-minimization evaluations are more complicated than cost descriptions because they aim to find the lowest cost alternative. They assume that the consequences of the alternatives are the same, or that the differences are unimportant. Examples of cost-minimization evaluations are of conventional or short-stay treatments, of comparable outcome drugs, of home and hospital treatment, of day compared to inpatient treatment and of private and public services. Like cost-description evaluations, cost minimization includes assumptions about costing inputs, but also assumptions about outcomes which may or may not be valid, even if previous RCTs have show insignificant differences in outcome.

The number and type of assumptions increase dramatically when we move to the next types of evaluation, and move from quantifying inputs to quantifying the consequences of an intervention, and then to comparing alternatives with different outcomes. For example, is the time of an unemployed person to be costed as the same as that of a highly paid person? What is the cost of suffering when waiting for a treatment (a 'non-resource use consequence')? How should we compare the value of a benefit now to receiving that benefit in five years' time – what 'discounting' formula should we use? This leads us to the three most well-known types of economic evaluations: cost-effectiveness, cost utility and cost-benefit.

Cost-effectiveness evaluations

Cost-effectiveness evaluations quantify both the costs of one or more interventions and the effects. These evaluations use one all-embracing measure of effect as a way of comparing alternatives – effects are often quantified in terms of number of lives saved, or life years or disability days which are gained or lost, or cases detected in a screening programme. Where only one measure of effect is used, it is easier to compare which of the alternatives has the greater effect on the one measure and to compare the costs of the alternatives for their different single effects. The art is to decide which single outcome measure most captures the value of the results of the intervention. We can see that some of the weaknesses of this approach are similar to those of experimental trials which concentrate on one measure of outcome.

An example is an early and famous Swedish evaluation of a drug to reduce cholesterol levels, which also builds on a randomized controlled trial (RCT) evaluation (SSSSG 1994). The RCT found in the experimental group 30 per cent less total mortality and 42 per cent less coronary mortality five years after the treatment (all patients in the trial already had heart disease). Jonsson's economic evaluation took life years gained as the measure of effect, and estimated how many fewer hospital days the treatment resulted in and the cost of this.

Taking these costs, and the lives saved (treating 100 patients with the drug for five years would save four deaths which would otherwise occur), he estimated that the cost of the treatment and the savings meant that each life year gained cost between US$6,500 and US$8,500. Note that, in this case, the costings do not include indirect costs, nursing home costs or effects other than mortality. Note also that in economic terms the decision whether or not to invest in the drug depends on a concept of an acceptable cost-effectiveness ratio – as a 'rule of thumb', one life year gained for less than $13,000 was at that time considered by some in Sweden as cost-effective.

Cost-effectiveness evaluations of services, educational programmes or policies, however, are rarely able to build on an RCT evaluation. Often we cannot be certain that the effects will result from the intervention. This is a particular problem for some non-treatment healthcare programmes such as health promotion schemes. However, economic evaluations are becoming more popular for interventions other than treatments. Managers and policy-makers increasingly need to know, in the precise terms that cost-effectiveness evaluations can give, the likely costs of the expected effects of new programmes or proposed changes. They need this information to justify starting or withdrawing programmes, and to face their more sophisticated critics who often already have cost-effectiveness information for similar interventions.

Cost-utility evaluations

Knowing that a treatment on average increases the quality of life by x years only allows crude comparisons between the treatment and another treatment or nothing. It does not allow comparisons between the quality of life produced by treatments, which are important comparisons to make in healthcare.

Cost-utility evaluations quantify the effects of an intervention in terms of how people value the effect, rather than in simple terms of lives or life years saved. The technical term for the value or usefulness of something to a person is 'utility'. Most cost-utility studies use one or more quality of life measures (Bowling 1992): the best-known measures of utility are the 'quality adjusted life year' (QALY) and the 'healthy day equivalent' (adjusted for quality of life).

Cost-utility evaluations allow comparisons across healthcare programmes, allowing us better to compare heart transplantation with ante-natal screening with smoking cessation programmes. We will see that some question the validity of these comparisons, but the point for the moment is that, in cost-effectiveness evaluations, comparisons are limited to treatments where the effectiveness measure can be meaningfully compared – number of lives saved is not alone a good outcome measure for comparing a liver transplantation programme with hospice care.

A cost-utility evaluation will do the following:

- calculate the cost of the interventions (or nothing);
- calculate the utility of the effects (how much value people give to the effect they get);
- then show how much it costs to get the effects for each intervention (or none).

The value of effects – for example, the value of being able to return to work three months earlier, or of being able to walk – are not thought up by the evaluators but are based on valuations made by ordinary people using special techniques. The simplest is nine boxes with box 1 = the 'worst imaginable health state' and box 9 = the 'best imaginable health state', or variations of this, such as a 'thermometer' with 100 = the best state and 0 = the worst. Another is the 'time trade-off': would you rather be healthy for five years and then die, or live for 15 years with, for example, less mobility and recurring pain (i.e. a defined sub-optimal health state)? If you have a clear preference to live longer, would this preference then apply to ten years, or seven? The aim is to find out the person's valuation of health states by reducing the time until the person has no preference between the alternatives.

A third method is the 'standard gamble', where a person is asked to choose between a state of poor health (which is defined) for x years, and a treatment which involves a chance of death or of being restored to full health. Would you rather not take the treatment if you had a 50 per cent chance of death? What about a 10 per cent chance? The chances are changed until the person is indifferent between the two alternatives. These and other techniques are summarized in Richardson (1992) and in more detail in Brooks (1986).

These techniques are of interest not just because they help us to understand some of the assumptions underlying cost-utility studies, but because they are methods which help people to express their personal valuations of different 'health states' and as such can be used in different types of evaluation. Knowing the value which people give to different health states helps clinicians and others to judge the value of an intervention and to make more informed decisions – and, to some extent, more democratic decisions.

Cost-utility evaluations using QALYs can compare the number of QALYs which could be expected if resources were used in different ways; or, expressed in a different way, the different costs to get one quality if the resources are used on different treatments. A very early report in 1990 illustrates this – from the SMAC (1990) report on cholesterol testing – an example of the kinds of comparison which can be made using this approach (Table 14.1).

These comparisons are only possible if you accept the assumptions and quantification methods underlying cost-utility evaluations, which are many (Hunter 1992; Smith 1992; Gerard and Mooney 1993). Criticisms of QALYs include: (1) that they are based on the values of small populations; (2) the small number of interventions which have

Table 14.1 Intervention and cost per QALY produced

Intervention	Cost per QALY produced (£)
Hospital haemodialysis for kidney failure	19,000
CABG (moderate, one vessel disease)	16,400
Cholesterol drug treatment	13,500
Heart transplant	6,700
Kidney transplant	4,000
CABG (main vessel disease)	1,090
Hip replacement	1,030
Cholesterol-lowering diet programme	176

Source: SMAC (1990).

been studied using this approach; (3) technical flaws; (4) a bias to giving greater value to duration of life than to life itself, and to valuing the young; (5) that QALYs do not distinguish between life-enhancing and life-saving treatments and try to equate them; and (6) the impact which QALY-based allocation would have on traditional rights of access to healthcare. Yet, without other information, these comparisons are increasingly being used to make resource allocation decisions. There is nothing wrong with doing so, as long as the assumptions and limitations are known and other information is also used.

Cost-benefit evaluations

You may remember hearing about compensation awards by law courts: to the farm-worker who lost his hand, or to a person who was still conscious during surgery. We may wonder how they judge these values: in fact, in non-jury cases there are detailed methods for 'fairly' calculating the value of a hand, or of a damaged business reputation. But how should we in the health services judge the monetary value of restoring health or function? How do economic evaluators assess the benefits and express these in money terms, as well as the costs of one or comparable interventions?

Cost-benefit economic evaluations quantify the effects of an intervention in monetary terms. Thus, rather than expressing the effects of a treatment as lives saved, or in quality of life units, the typical cost-benefit evaluation expresses the effects in terms of money value. These evaluations show that spending x money will result in benefits worth y money, and give an easily understood idea of the 'value for money' of the intervention.

For example, in late 1989, the Swedish National Road Administration calculated the cost of different measures to reduce road accidents and compared these costs to their average 'cost per casualty' for a fatality (US$550,000 total, which includes US$60,000 for healthcare costs, net loss of a worker's production, and 'costs owing to property damage and administration', plus US$490,000 as 'human value' costs (i.e. 'non-resource use consequences')). The reader will be comforted to know that the costs of 'severe casualty' are about one-seventh of these costs (in 1989 values).

Both inputs and the outputs are quantified in the same (monetary) terms. Cost-benefit evaluations also make it possible to compare the value of the effects of different interventions in monetary terms. This involves assumptions that different effects can be quantified and reduced to the same unit of money value.

Would you pay for a helicopter ambulance service?

'How much would your household be willing to contribute each year in taxes to a helicopter ambulance service?' This question comes from an early Norwegian study which used a technique that is being explored as an alternative to QALYs for measuring the benefits of healthcare: the 'willingness to pay' technique (Olsen and Donaldson 1993). The aim is to get people to say how much they would be prepared to pay for a particular treatment or service, which is described together with its benefits and risks, usually assuming that they would pay through taxation. The advantages are that people use a familiar unit of measure – money – and bring into their valuation of the intervention a sense of what they would have to give up by not having the money. The more complicated versions of this technique ask how much people would pay for a number of services. In the study cited, people at that time in Norway were, in fact, prepared to pay significantly more for helicopters and heart operations than for hip replacements. While this method for quantifying benefit in money terms does make greater use of ordinary people's valuation, the techniques used are not without problems (Olsen and Donaldson 1993).

Box 14.1 Definition of types of economic evaluation

- *Cost description*: measurement of the costs of one thing, or of more than one, in a way which allows an explicit or implicit comparison of costs. (A 'partial' evaluation looks at only one intervention and does not make an explicit comparison.)
- *Cost minimization*: assumes that the differences in outcome produced by the alternatives are not significant, and calculates the cost of each alternative with the purpose of discovering which is the lowest cost.
- *Cost-effectiveness*: the effectiveness or consequences as shown on one measure, for the cost (e.g. lives saved, cases of diseases avoided or years of healthy life). No attempt is made to value the consequences – it is assumed that the output is of value. Used to compare the different costs of using different ways to achieve the same end result.
- *Cost utility*: considers the utility of the end result to the patient for the cost. Often uses the QALY measure, where extended life is at the expense of side effects. Measures consequences in time units adjusted by health utility weights (i.e. states of health associated with outcome are valued relative to each other). More complex than cost-effectiveness.
- *Cost-benefit*: an attempt to value the consequences of a programme in money terms, so as to compare the assessed value with the actual costs. A range of benefits are valued in money terms. Concerned with how worthwhile an end result is for the cost.

Cost-benefit evaluation methods are also used to assess interventions to organization and for investment appraisals of proposed building or service schemes. An example is the evaluation of health information technology (HIT) systems: cost-benefit analyses can be carried out to predict the costs and benefits of a system, or retrospectively to evaluate the actual costs and benefits. However, economic evaluations of

HIT systems, like evaluations of other types of intervention to organization, face problems in isolating the effects of the system from other changes which might have occurred. There are also the familiar problems of defining what is in 'the box' – is the HIT intervention the hardware, or the training as well? In many cases, the HIT system does not just automate a manual system, but changes the whole way work is carried out. Neither the intervention nor the context is likely to be stable (Keen 1994).

Strengths and weaknesses of economic evaluations

It is important to distinguish the strengths and weaknesses of the economic perspective in general from the different strengths and weaknesses of each type of economic evaluation. Criticisms of QALYs are not criticisms of the economic perspective, or of types of evaluation such as a cost-minimization study. This chapter aimed to give an impression of how the economic perspective is applied in evaluation, and of some of the assumptions of different types of economic evaluations. Not all economic analy-ses are evaluations, but most are because they involve an explicit comparison, or the implicit comparison of the 'do nothing' opportunity cost: describing the resources used – often in money terms – invites us to think of other ways of spending the money.

All economic evaluations attribute value to an intervention by using systematically gained information about the resources used, and by comparing the intervention to nothing at all or to other uses of resources. Many also gather information about effects and use outcome measures to measure effectiveness or benefit. Many assess effects other than those for the patient, but studies differ in the scope of their effects assessments and in whether they take a health service or societal perspective. Economic evaluations differ in how narrowly they define costs and benefits, and in the accuracy and the validity of their measures. The purpose of most economic evaluations is to compare the cost-benefit or utility of the intervention with other uses of the finance. Some meta-studies draw together a number of evaluations of the same intervention to produce a synthesis evaluation, but there are technical problems in combining studies in this way.

From an economic perspective, healthcare funders have to maximize the benefit they can get from the total sum they have to spend. They need information about costs, and about outcome performance to decide benefits, and this information needs to be about both national averages and potential local providers. Buxton (1992) proposes that funders should only finance 'new' treatments on condition that the provider evaluates them, and that funders should be prepared to contribute to the cost of evaluation.

Economic evaluations are often combined with, or built on, experimental evaluations. The economic analysis may be perfect, but any weaknesses in the experimental design will invalidate any practical conclusions (HERG 1996). Economic evaluations, in common with other types of evaluations which express results in quantitative terms, may give an impression of objectivity which is not justified, and which can mislead even experts. There are many assumptions about how to quantify costs, including which costs to exclude from the calculations. There are assumptions about how to quantify health consequences for individuals (e.g. just years of life or quality of life, and which aspects of quality?), about when to measure consequences and about which consequences to exclude (e.g. effects on relatives, costs for other services). There are assumptions about how to make valid comparisons of the effects of intervention when the effects of each intervention are expressed in the same units, such as quality of life units.

Where there is no other basis for resource allocation decisions, managers and politicians are increasingly using cost-utility or other economic analyses. Few detailed cost-utility evaluations have been carried out on interventions other than treatments, in part because economic evaluators have tended to develop methods which focus on individuals, such as utility to individuals. There is great scope for applying utility quantification and costing to interventions such as health promotion and educational programmes for patients, citizens and healthcare workers. (Three early papers in one volume of *Health Education Research* consider the role of health economics in the evaluation of health promotion (e.g. Craig and Walker 1996), and Haycox (1994) describes a methodology for estimating costs and benefits.) The fact that many economic evaluations have concentrated on the costs to health services and on individual-based valuations does not mean that the perspective cannot take a societal view. As we increasingly consider the many influences other than health services on health, and seek the cooperation of other sectors to improve health, we should also consider the social costs and benefits of health treatments, services and policies in judging their value.

Whatever the drawbacks, the discipline of economic evaluation, like that of experimental evaluation, directly confronts many issues and involves assumptions which arise in most types of evaluation. Even if an evaluator or a user of evaluation is not involved in an economic evaluation, it is important that he or she understands issues such as those involved in quantifying resources and consequences and is aware of the detailed and through examination which health economists have given to these issues.

Most evaluators need to give a description of the resources used by the item which they evaluate. They also need to describe in their proposal how much resource the study they propose will use and the costs, as well as expected benefits and possibly savings, that could result from the evaluation. Will it ultimately be a 'cost-free evaluation'? The theories developed by economists about how to quantify resources, and criticisms of the methods economists use, need to be understood by all evaluators and users of evaluations.

Conclusion

Economic evaluations help others to judge the value of an intervention by gathering information about the resources consumed by an intervention, expressed as costs. Many also gather information about the consequences of the intervention. Some economic evaluations will only consider a limited set of resources, for example, those consumed by one health service and those which are easily calculated. Others take a broader view of the resources consumed, show costs to society and note 'difficult to quantify' costs. Full economic evaluations quantify the consequences of an intervention as well as the costs, and also compare two or more alternatives, even though one alternative may be the 'do nothing' option or a placebo. Common types of economic evaluation are:

- Cost-description and cost-minimization evaluations: these describe only the costs of the intervention.
- Cost-effectiveness studies: use one measure of effectiveness, such as lives saved, and compare the cost and effectiveness of interventions.
- Cost-utility evaluations assess the utility or value of health states produced by different interventions for the cost. They allow comparison of different interventions used in different health services.
- Cost-benefit studies: they value both the resources consumed and the consequences of an intervention in money terms, thus allowing easy value for money judgements.

All economic evaluations make technical and value assumptions when they quantify costs and consequences. These are usually stated, but are sometimes only understandable to economists: for non-economists, the precise quantification may give the impression that the findings are entirely objective, and that there are no judgements of value underlying the study.

Glossary

Action research: a systematic investigation which aims to contribute to knowledge as well as solve a practical problem.

Audit: an investigation into whether an activity meets explicit standards as defined by an auditing document. The auditing process can be carried by external auditors or internally for self-review, and can use external ready-made audit standards or internally developed standards. Medical and clinical audits use pre-existing standards or setting standards, comparing practice with standards, and changing practice if necessary, and are usually carried out internally for self-review and improvement. Peer-audit can use already-existing standards, or practitioners can develop their own, but usually practitioners adapt existing standards to their own situation.

Blinding:

- *Single-blinded trail*: the people in the control and experimental groups (subjects) do not know which group they are in.
- *Double-blinded trail*: neither the subjects nor the service providers know which group is the experimental and which is the control.

The 'box': the boundary around the intervention, which defines what is evaluated, and separates it from the environment. Includes inside the box a specification of the components of the intervention.

Budget impact analysis (BIA): Predicts how a change will impact the spending and savings over time of a defined budget holder. It can be used for budget planning, forecasting and for computing the impact of health technology changes on premiums in health insurance schemes (Mauskopf et al. 2007).

Business case: One definition shows that 'business case' includes ROI, but is broader:

> A business case for a health improvement intervention exists if the entity that invests in the intervention realizes a financial return on its investment in a reasonable time frame, using a reasonable rate of discounting. This may be realized in bankable dollars (profit), a reduction in losses for a given program or population, or avoided costs. In addition, a business case may exist if the investing entity believes that a positive indirect effect on organizational function and sustainability will accrue within a reasonable time frame.
>
> (Leatherman et al. 2003, p. 18)

Case control study: a retrospective observational study of people or organizations with a particular characteristic ('cases') compared to those which do not have this characteristic (controls), to find out possible causes or influences which could explain the characteristic.

Case study: 'attempts to examine a contemporary phenomenon in its real-life context, especially when the boundaries between context and phenomenon are not clearly evident' (Yin 1981).

Cohort: a group of people, usually sharing one or more characteristics, who are followed over time to find out what happens to them.

Confounding factors or variables: something other than the intervention which could influence the measured outcome.

Continuous quality improvement: an approach for ensuring that staff continually improve work processes by using proven quality methods to discover and resolve the causes of quality problems in a systematic way.

Control group or control site: a group of people or an organization which do not receive the intervention. The evaluation compares them to the experimental group or site, which gets the intervention. People are randomly allocated to either group, or, if this is not possible, the control group or site is 'matched' with the experimental group.

Cost-benefit: valuing the consequences of a programme in money terms, so as to compare the assessed value with the actual costs. A range of benefits are valued in money terms.

Cost description: measurement of the costs of one thing, or of more than one, in a way that allows an explicit or implicit comparison of costs. (A 'partial' economic evaluation looks at only one intervention and does not make an explicit comparison.)

Cost-effectiveness: the effectiveness or consequences as shown on one measure, for the cost (e.g. lives saved, cases of diseases avoided, or years of healthy life). No attempt is made to value the consequences – it is assumed that the output is of value. Used to compare the different costs of using different ways to achieve the same end result.

Cost minimization: assumes that the differences in outcome produced by the alternatives are not significant, and calculates the cost of each alternative with the purpose of discovering which is the lowest cost.

Cost Savings Spreading Agency (CSSA): An independent agency providing investment finance, monitoring improvement and savings and ensuring savings and cost of an improvement are fairly distributed.

Cost utility: considers the utility of the end result to the patient for the cost. Often uses the QALY measure. Measures consequences in time units adjusted by health utility weights (i.e. states of health associated with outcome are valued relative to each other). More complex than cost-effectiveness.

- **Cost of the problem**: Cost of the providers' poor-quality performance to the provider (and to other stakeholders) (e.g. cost of infections which are potentially preventable, such as 3 per cent ICU central line infection rate).

- **Savings or loss**: How much the provider saves or loses, taking into account the spend cost of the improvement, at one year, three years and five years (and for other stakeholders).
- **Spend cost**: Investment cost to reduce the problem by 20 per cent and 50 per cent to the provider (and other stakeholders) (e.g. cost to implement central line care practice bundle).
- **Time to pay back**: From the start of the spending, how many months before savings pay back the spend cost, if they ever do? (E.g. savings begin at six months after investment starts for ICU central line care practice bundle, but savings need to add up for nine months to pay off the investment.)

Criterion: a comparison against which we judge the intervention – effectiveness is an example often of such a criterion.

Efficiency:

- **Horizontal target efficiency**: the extent to which the service reaches all those who need it.
- **Input mix efficiency**: the extent to which the mix of care inputs reflects costs – we can improve input mix efficiency by substituting lower-cost labour.
- **Market efficiency (or output mix efficiency)**: the degree to which the outputs of a service reflect consumer preferences.
- **Technical efficiency**: the amount produced for the input (input/output).
- **Vertical target efficiency**: whether the service is targeted to those most in need.

Evaluated: the action or intervention which is evaluated – the subject of the evaluation.

Evaluation: judging the value of something by gathering information about it in a systematic way and by making a comparison, for the purpose of making a better-informed decision.

Evaluation-informed management (EIM): making more informed management decisions by using research evidence and evidence from inside the organization, and making more effective actions and projects by using evaluation concepts to plan management interventions.

Evaluator: the person doing the evaluation.

Evidence-based medicine:

> The conscientious, explicit, and judicious use of current best evidence in making decisions about the care of individual patients. The practice of EBM means integrating individual clinical expertise with best available external clinical evidence from systematic research.
>
> (Sackett et al. 1996)

External evaluators: research or consultancy units not directly managed by and independent from the sponsor and user of the evaluation.

Indicator: a quantitative measurement that produces data that are comparable.

Internal evaluators: evaluation and development units which are internal to the organization, which evaluate treatments services or policies carried out by the organization or one of its divisions.

Intervention: an action on, or attempt to change a person, population or organization, which is the subject of an evaluation (e.g. a health service, programme, policy or reform).

ISO 9000: a description of how an organization should write down in a quality manual ('documentation') its arrangements for allocating responsibility for quality, how it should define objectives, policies and procedures, and how the organization then ensures that these arrangements are followed (control) and poor quality is recorded. ISO 9000 is a 'standard' for a 'quality system'.

Matching: ensuring that people (or organizations) in the experimental and control groups (or sites) are the same, in all the characteristics which could affect the outcome of the intervention which is given to the experimental group or site.

Monetizable value improvement (MVI): A value improvement which easily provides additional cash or savings in the end of the year budget. A change which saves money *and* improves quality (e.g. the ICU can treat more patients and get paid extra for this because there are fewer days spent treating infections).

Monitoring: continuous supervision of an activity to check whether plans and procedures are being followed. (Audit is a sub-type of the wider activity of monitoring.)

Operationalize: converting something general (e.g. a criterion) into something specific, usually into something which we can measure (e.g. a measure of amount of sleep such as a diary record).

Organizational audit: an external inspection of aspects of a service, in comparison to established standards, and a review of an organization's arrangements to control and assure the quality of its products or services. Audits use criteria (or 'standards') against which auditors judge elements of a service's planning, organization, systems and performance.

Outcome: the difference an intervention makes to the person, population, or organization which is the target of the intervention.

Outcome measure: a measure of an important predicted effect of the intervention on the target person or population.

Patient pathway: a description and diagram of the series of steps over time taken by a patient passing to and through different services when seeking help for a health problem (Øvretveit 1993). The pathway may be a simple diagrams of decisions at different stages (patient flow diagram), or it may be a more detailed checklist and record of tasks to be done at different stages (e.g. critical path; integrated care pathway, anticipated recovery path, care plan, care protocols, care paths). Pathways are often defined for patients with a particular type of health condition or diagnosis where their care is predictable and standardization can reduce unwanted variations in care.

Placebo: something which the subjects of the intervention think is an intervention, but which has no known 'active ingredient' (used to control for effects which may be caused only by subjects thinking that they are receiving an intervention). Means 'to please'.

Police car effect: people who think they are being evaluated follow regulations more closely than when they think that they are not being evaluated.

Procedure/protocol: a written statement of how to carry out a task. Some procedures give more details about a part of the patient's pathway or part of a process. Some procedures are written by referring to research into effective ways to carry out a treatment (evidence-based procedures/protocols or guidelines).

Process: A sequence of activities that produces a valued change in a person, object or information.

Proportional improvement: The spend cost of the improvement is proportional to the benefits achieved either in savings or in higher quality or both.

Prospective evaluation: designing an evaluation and then collecting data while the intervention is happening, and usually also before and after the intervention.

Public health quality: the ability of a health system to protect and improve the health of a population. It depends on traditional improvements to healthcare services, but also on programmes for those who make little use of these services and whose voice is rarely heard in surveys.

Qualificiency: using the fewest resources to consistently achieve a standard of care, which meets patients' essential health needs and wants.

Quality: meeting the health needs of those most in need at the lowest cost, and within regulations (Øvretveit 1992).

Quality accreditation: a certification through an external evaluation of whether a practitioner, equipment or a service meets standards which are thought to contribute to quality processes and outcomes.

Quality assurance: a general term for activities and systems for monitoring and improving quality. Quality assurance involves, but is more than measuring quality and evaluating quality.

Quality-cost return on investment (QCROI): The amount of time and money saved by the value improvement, expressed as a ratio of the spend cost to the savings at years 1, 3, 5. (A 'business case' analysis does not consider evidence of quality, and some health economics research does not provide evidence of quality improvement.)

Quality problem: an invitation to close the gap between what is, and how things could be, in order to be better.

Quality programme: a set of activities to ensure and develop the quality of a service, which are usually planned and organization-wide, and include training, providing quality methods expertise, setting up project teams, defining responsibilities for quality and measuring quality.

Quality project: a time-limited task to solve a quality problem or improve quality, undertaken by a specially created team using quality methods in a structured way.

Quality system: a set of requirements which state the actions a healthcare organization must take to systematically identify and correct quality problems. Many quality systems require the organization to define responsibilities for quality and the necessary procedures, to ensure these are known to all personnel and that quality performance is documented and corrective action is taken when poor quality occurs. A quality system is a coordinated set of procedures, division of responsibilities, and processes for setting quality standards and procedures, identifying quality problems and resolving these problems. (BSI 5750 and ISO 9000 are standards for a quality system.)

Randomization: allocating people in a random way to an experimental or a control group. The purpose is to try to ensure that the people (or organizations) with characteristics which might affect the outcome are allocated evenly to both groups. This is because there are many known and unknown characteristics which may influence outcome. Randomization allows the evaluators to consider any differences between the two groups which are more than chance differences as significant and avoids the need for matching.

Randomized controlled trial: an experiment where one group gets the intervention and another group does not, and people are assigned to both groups in a random way.

Research – basic or pure: the use of scientific methods which are appropriate for discovering valid knowledge of a phenomenon for the purpose of contributing to scientific knowledge about the subject.

Retrospective evaluation: looking into the past for evidence about the intervention.

Review: a single or regular assessment of an activity, which may or may not compare the activity to an explicit plan, criteria or standards. (Most audits or monitoring are types of review. Many 'managerial evaluations' are reviews or monitoring.)

Self-evaluation: practitioners or teams who evaluate their own practice so as to improve it.

Sensitivity: the ability of a test to detect all true positives, or of a measure to detect changes in the phenomena being measured.

Specificity: the ability of a test to identify true negatives.

Sponsor: one who initiates or pays for the evaluation.

Stakeholder: a person or group with interests in the outcome of an intervention or an evaluation of it (e.g. patients, citizens, health personnel, managers). Stakeholders in value improvement are: patients, providers (individuals and services), funders, regulators. Those who may benefit from the value improvement, and who may need to spend or change to achieve the improvement.

System: a set of elements, which interact with each other, and which function as a whole, to produce an effect. Systems thinking is seeing the connections: seeing that the causes of quality problems are not one thing, but how different things interact, and seeing the solutions as changing interactions and how the whole works, not changing one thing. Systems management is creating connections and synergy through synchronizing.

System of care quality: the ability of a set of services, which a patient needs, to cooperate to assess and meet the requirements of the patient, at the lowest costs, without duplication or errors and in a way in which the patient experiences care as one continuous episode.

System of care quality development: combining professional, management and organizational quality methods to develop the 'system of care' experienced by the patient to produce better patient experiences and less patient suffering using fewer resources.

Target: the part or whole of the person or population which the intervention aims to have an effect on.

Total quality management (TQM): a comprehensive strategy of organizational and attitude change to enable staff to learn and use quality methods in order to reduce costs and meet the requirements of patients and other 'customers'. Quality is 'a method of management'– quality is determined by systems of care, and management are responsible for the performance of these systems.

User: those who make use of or act on an evaluation.

Validity: external validity: the ability of an evaluation experiment to show that the findings would also apply if the intervention is applied in another setting.

Validity: internal validity: the validity of an evaluation experiment, for example in being able to show whether or not the intervention has an effect or the size of the effect.

Value criterion: what is important to people in how they judge the value of an intervention.

Value improvement (VI): An intervention for which there is evidence of both improved quality for the patient *and* less waste or better use of resources (e.g. changing care practices reduces infections in ICU).

Variable:

- **Dependent variable**: the outcome or end result of a treatment service or policy. (The main thing the evaluation has to discover, e.g. lower blood pressure, nurses follow a procedure after receiving an educational intervention.)
- **Independent variable**: something which may cause the outcome. Any variable whose effect on another variable is to be assessed.

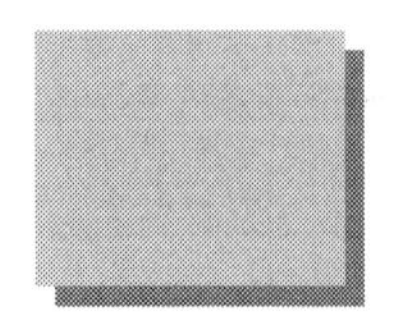

References

Academy Health (2012) *Using Evidence to Build a Learning Health Care System, Research Insights*. Academy Health 2012. Available at: www.academyhealth.org/files/publications/AHUsingEvidence2012.pdf? (accessed 2 January 2014).

Adamou, B. (2013) *Guide for Monitoring Scale-up of Health Practices and Interventions: MEASURE Evaluation Population and Reproductive Health (PRH)*. Available at: https://www.cpc.unc.edu/measure/prh (accessed 4 January 2014).

Ader, M., Berensson, K., Carlsson, P., Granath, M. and Urwitz, V. (2001) Quality indicators for health promotion programmes, *Health Promotion International*, 16(2): 187–95.

AHRQ (2011) Unit-based safety program improves safety culture, reduces medication errors and length of stay, report from AHRQ Innovations Exchange. Available at: http://www.ahrq.gov/.

Alexander, J.A., Weiner, B.J., Shortell, S.M., Baker, L.C. and Becker, M.P. (2006) The role of organizational infrastructure in implementation of hospitals' quality improvement, *Hosp Top*, 84(1): 11–20.

Altman, D (1991) *Practical Statistics for Medical Research*. London: Chapman & Hall.

Ammenwertha, E., Brenderb, J., Nykänenc, P., Ulrich Prokosch, D.H., Rigbye, M. and Talmond, J. (2004) Visions and strategies to improve evaluation of health information systems: reflections and lessons based on the HIS-EVAL workshop, *Innsbruck International Journal of Medical Informatics*, 73(6): 479–91.

Anker, M., Guidotti, R.J., Orzeszyna, S., Sapirie, S.A. and Thuriaux, M.C. (1993) Rapid evaluation methods (REM) of health services performance: methodological observations, *Bulletin of World Health Organization*, 71(1): 15–21.

Apodaca, A. (2013) Defining your research questions and hypotheses. Available at: http://science.dodlive.mil/2010/10/04/defining-the-beginning-importance-of-research-questions-hypotheses/ (accessed 21 January 2013).

ARCH (2014) *Applied Research Collaboration for Health*. Available at: http://archcanada.ipower.com/?page_id=2 (accessed 4 January 2014).

Ash, A., Fienberg, S., Louis, T., Normand, S., Stukel, T. and Utts, J. (2012) *Statistical Issues in Assessing Hospital Performance*. Washington, DC: The COPSS-CMS White Paper Committee, CMS.

Astra, J. and Littlejohn, A. (1993) Doll therapy worsens depression by raising expectations, *Journal of Pharmaceutical Ethics*, 2(4): 13–14.

Barnes, M., Matka, E. and Sullivan, H. (2003) Evidence, understanding and complexity: evaluation in non-linear systems, *Evaluation*, 9(3): 265–84.

Beecher, H.K. (1955) The powerful placebo, *Journal of the American Medical Association*, 159: 1602–6.

Begg, C., Cho, M., Eastwood, S., Horton, R., Moher, D., Olkin, I., et al. (1996) Improving the quality of reporting of randomized controlled trials. The CONSORT statement. *JAMA*, 276: 637–9.

Benning, A., Ghaleb, M., Suokas, A., Dixon-Woods, M., Dawson, J., Barber, N., et al. (2011)

Large-scale organisational intervention to improve patient safety in four UK hospitals: mixed method evaluation, *BMJ*. Online: doi:10.1136/bmj.d195.

Benson, H. and Epstein, M.D. (1975) The placebo effect: a neglected asset in the care of patients, *Journal of the American Medical Association*, 232: 1225–7.

Benson, H. and McCallie, D.P., Jr. (1979) Angina pectoris and the placebo effect, *New England Journal of Medicine*, 300: 1424–9.

Berwick, D. (2008) The science of improvement, *JAMA*, 299: 1182–4.

Berwick, D.M., Calkins, D.R., McCannon, C.J. and Hackbarth, A.D. (2006) The 100,000 lives campaign: setting a goal and a deadline for improving health care quality, *JAMA*, 295(3): 324–7.

Bickman, K. (2008) The science of quality improvement (letter to the editor) *JAMA*, 300(4): 391.

Bickman, L. (ed.) (1987) Using program theory in program evaluation, vol. 33 of *New Directions in Program Evaluation*. San Francisco: Jossey-Bass.

Blaise, P. and Kegels, G. (2004) A realistic approach to the evaluation of the quality management movement in health care systems: a comparison between European and African contexts based on Mintzberg's organizational models, *International Journal of Health Planning Management*, 19: 337–64.

Booth, A. and Falzon, F. (2001) Evaluating information service innovations in the health service: 'If I was planning on going there I wouldn't start from here', *Health Information Journal*, 7: 13–19.

Boutron, I., Moher, D., Altman, D., Schulz, D. and Ravaud, P. and CONSORT Group (2008) Methods and processes of the CONSORT Group: example of an extension for trials assessing nonpharmacologic treatments, *Annals of International Medicine*, 148(4):W-60–W-66. doi:10.7326/0003-4819-148-4-200802190-00008-w1.

Bowling, A. (1992) *Measuring Health: A Review of Quality of Life Measures*. Milton Keynes: Open University Press.

Brennan, S., Bosch, M., Buchan, H. and Green, S. (2012) Measuring organizational and individual factors thought to influence the success of quality improvement in primary care: a systematic review of instruments, *Implementation Science*, 7:121. doi:10.1186/1748-5908-7-121.

Brooks, R. (1986) *Scaling in Health Status Measurement*. Lund: The Swedish Institute of Health Economics.

Brown, C.A. and Lilford, R.J. (2006) The stepped wedge trial design: a systematic review, *BMC Medical Research Methodology*, 6.

Brown, W., Yen, P., Rojas, M. and Schnall, R. (2013) Assessment of the Health IT Usability Evaluation Model (Health-ITUEM) for evaluating mobile health (mHealth) technology, *Journal of Biomedical Informatics*. Available at: HONF 2013 Health On the Net Foundation Standards. www.HealthOnNet.org (accessed 21 November 2013).

Brycea, J., Victora, C., Boerma, T., Peters, D. and Black, R. (2010) *Evaluating the Scale-Up for Maternal and Child Survival: A Common Framework*. Baltimore, MD: Institute for International Programs, Bloomberg School of Public Health.

Buxton, M. (1992) Scarce resources and informed choices, AMI conference paper, HERG, Brunel University, November.

Byng, R., Norman, I. and Redfern, S. (2005) Using realistic evaluation to evaluate a practice-level intervention to improve primary healthcare for patients with long-term mental illness, *Evaluation*, 11(1): 69–93.

Byng, R., Norman, I., Redfern, S. and Jones, R. (2008) Exposing the key functions of a complex intervention for shared care in mental health: case study of a process evaluation, *BMC Health Services Research*, 8: 274.

Campbell. M., Fitzpatrick, R., Haines, A., Kinmouth, A.L., Sandercock, P., Spiegelhalter, D., et al. (2000) Framework for design and evaluation of complex interventions to improve health. *BMJ*, 321: 694–6.

Cantrell, C.R., Eaddy, M.T. and Shah, M.B. (2006) Methods for evaluating patient adherence to antidepressant therapy, *Medical Care*, 44(4): 300–3.

Carey, R. and Lloyd, R. (1995) *Measuring Quality Improvement in Healthcare*. New York: Quality Resources.

Cartwright, M., Hirani, S.P., Rixon, L., Beynon, M., Doll, H., et al. (2013) Whole systems demonstrator evaluation team: effect of telehealth on quality of life and psychological outcomes over 12 months: nested study of patient reported outcomes in a pragmatic, cluster randomised controlled trial, *BMJ*, Feb 26: 346:f653. doi: 10.1136/bmj.f653.

CDC (2008) Evaluation brief: logic model. Available at: http://www.cdc.gov/healthyyouth/evaluation/index.htm (accessed 26 March 2014).

Choudhry, N., Fletcher, R. and Soumerai, S. (2005) Systematic review: the relationship between clinical experience and quality of health care, *Annals of International Medicine*, 142: 260–73.

Coleman, E., Parry, C., Chalmers, S. and Min, S.J. (2006) The care transitions intervention: results of a randomized controlled trial, *Archives of International Medicine*, 166: 1822–8.

Commonwealth Fund (2013) Hospital comparison website. Available at: http://www.whynot-thebest.org/ (accessed 21 December 2013).

Concato, J. and Horwitz, R.I. (2004) Beyond randomised versus observational studies, *Lancet*, 363(9422):1660–1.

Concato, J., Lawler, E.V., Lew, R.A., Gaziano, J.M., Aslan, M. and Huang, G.D. (2010) Observational methods in comparative effectiveness research, *American Journal of Medicine*, 123(12) (suppl. 1): e16–e23.

Coyte, P.C. and Holmes, D. (2007) Health care technology adoption and diffusion in a social context, *Policy, Politics & Nursing Practice*, 8: 47–54.

Craig, N. and Walker, D. (1996) Choice and accountability in health promotion: the role of health economics, *Health Education Research*, 11(3): 355–60.

Craig, P. et al. (2008) *Developing and Evaluating Complex Interventions: New Guidance*. London: Medical Research Council. Available at: www.mrc.ac.uk/ (accessed January 2014).

Craig, P., Dieppe, P., et al. (2008) Developing and evaluating complex interventions: the new Medical Research Council guidance, *BMJ*, 337:a1655. ID Number 1047. Available at: http://www.ncbi.nlm.nih.gov/entrez.

Craig, P., Macintyre, S., Michie, S., Nazareth, I. and Petticrew, M. (2006) *Developing and Evaluating Complex Interventions: New Guidance*. London: MRC. Available at: www.mrc.ac.uk/complexinterventionsguidance (accessed 15 December 2013).

Damberg, C., Sorbero, M., Lovejoy, S., Lauderdale, K., Wertheimer, S., Smith, A., Waxman, D. and Schnyer, C. (2011) An evaluation of the use of performance, in *Measures in Health Care*. Santa Monica, CA: RAND. Available at: http://www.rand.org/ (accessed 4 January 2014).

Davis, P. (2005) The limits of realist evaluation: surfacing and exploring assumptions in assessing the best value performance regime, *Evaluation*, 11(3): 275–95.

Davis, P., Milne, B., Parker, K., Hider, P., Lay-Yee, R., Cumming, J., et al. (2013) Efficiency, effectiveness, equity (E3): evaluating hospital performance in three dimensions. *Health Policy*, 112. Available at: http://dx.doi.org/10.1016/j.healthpol (accessed 2 August 2013).

Devon, E., Hinton, D., Chhean, D., Pich, V., et al. (2005) A randomized controlled trial of cognitive-behavior therapy for Cambodian refugees with treatment-resistant PTSD and panic attacks: a cross-over design, *Journal of Traumatic Stress*, 18(6): 617–29.

Dixon-Woods, M., Bosk, C., Aveling, E., Goeschel, C. and Pronovost, P. (2011) Explaining

Michigan: developing an ex post theory of a quality improvement program, *The Milbank Quarterly*, 89(2): 167–205.

Dodd, M.J. (1982) Assessing patient self-care for side effects of cancer chemotherapy: Part I, *Cancer Nursing*, 5(6): 447–51.

Dreyer, N.A, Tunis, S.R., Berger, M., et al. (2010) Why observational studies should be among the tools used in comparative effectiveness research, *Health Affairs*, (Millwood), 29: 1818e25.

Dr Foster (2014) The hospital guide. Available at: http://drfosterintelligence.co.uk/thought-leadership/hospital-guide/ (accessed 4 January 2014).

Drummond, M., Stoddard, G. and Torrence, G. (1987) *Methods for the Economic Evaluation of Health Care Programmes*. Oxford: Oxford Medical Publications.

EFQM (European Foundation for Quality Management) (1999) *The Excellence Model*, Brussels: EFQM.

Eisenstein, E.L., Juzwishin, D., Kushniruk, A.W. and Nahm, M. (2011) Defining a framework for health information technology evaluation, *Studies in Health Technology and Informatics*, 164: 94–9.

Ekberg, K. et al. (1994) Controlled two-year follow-up of rehabilitation for disorders in the neck and shoulders, *Occupational and Environmental Medicine*, 51: 833–8.

EPOC (2009) Cochrane Effective Practice and Organisation of Care Group. Available at: http://www.epoc.cochrane.org/en/authors.html.

Etheredge, L. (2007) A rapid-learning health system, *Health Affairs*. Web Exclusive w107-118. DOI 10.1377/hlthaff.26.2.w107 (accessed 4 January 2014).

Fan, E., Laupacis, A., Pronovost, P., et al. (2010) How to use an article about quality improvement, *JAMA*, 304(20): 2279– 87.

Fawcett, L. et al. (1997) In I. Rootman and D. McQueen (eds) *Evaluating Health Promotion Approaches*. Copenhagen: WHO.

Ferlie, E., Fitzgerald, L., Wood, M. and Hawkins, C. (2005) The non-spread of innovations: the mediating role of professionals. *Academy of Management Journal*, 48: 117–34.

Flottorp, S., Havelsrud, K. and Oxman, A.D. (2003) Process evaluation of a cluster randomized trial of tailored interventions to implement guidelines in primary care: why is it so hard to change practice?, *Family Practice*, 20: 333–9.

Francisco, V., Paine, A. and Fawcett, S. (1993) A methodology for monitoring and evaluating community health coalitions, *Health Education Research*, 8: 403–16.

Franklin, B. (1941) Letter to John Pringle (1757). In I. Cohen (ed.) *Benjamin Franklin's Experiments*. Cambridge, MA: Harvard University Press.

Freemantle, N., Nazareth, I., Eccles, M., Wood, J., Haines, A. and the EBOR Trialists (2002) A randomised trial of the effect of educational outreach by community pharmacists on prescribing in primary care, *British Journal of General Practice*, 52: 290–5.

Friedman, C.P., Wong, A.K. and Blumenthal, D. (2010) Achieving a nationwide learning health system, *Science Translational Medicine*, 2.

Friedman, C.P. and Wyatt, J.C. (2006) *Evaluation Methods in Bio-Medical Informatics*, 2nd edn. New York: Springer-Verlag.

Friedman, L.M., Furberg, C.D. and DeMets, D.L. (1998) *Fundamentals of Clinical Trials*, 3rd edn. New York: Springer.

Ganann, R., Ciliska, D. and Thomas, H. (2010) Expediting systematic reviews: methods and implications of rapid reviews, *Implementation Science*, 5:56. Available at: http://www.implementationscience.com/content/5/1/56 (accessed 21 January 2013).

GAVI (2011) Monitoring and Evaluation Framework and Strategy, 2011–2015, Monitoring and Evaluation Working Group of the International Health Partnership and related initiatives

(IHP+). Available at: www.gavialliance.org/library/documents/gavi-documents/strategy (accessed 4 January 2014).

Gerard, K. and Mooney, G. (1993) QALY league tables: handle with care, *Health Economics*, 2: 59–64.

Glasgow, R.E., Lichtenstein, E. and Marcus, A.C. (2003) Why don't we see more translation of health promotion research to practice? Rethinking the efficacy to effectiveness transition, *American Journal of Public Health*, 93:1261–7.

Glasziou, P., Meats, E., Heneghan, C. and Shepperd, S. (2008) What is missing from descriptions of treatment in trials and reviews?, *BMJ*, 336: 1472–4.

Goetz, M., Bowman, C., Hoang, T., Anaya, H., Osborn, T., Gifford., A. and Asch, S. (2008) Implementing and evaluating a regional strategy to improve testing rates in VA patients at risk for HIV, utilizing the QUERI process as a guiding framework: QUERI Series, *Implementation Science*, 3(16). Online. doi: 10.1186/1748-5908-3-16.

Gold, M., Helms, D. and Guterman, S. (2011) Identifying, monitoring, and assessing promising innovations: using evaluation to support rapid- cycle change, Issue Brief, Washington, DC: The Commonwealth Fund, publication 1512, vol. 12.

Green, L. and Glasgow, R. (2006) Evaluating the relevance, generalization, and applicability of research: issues in external validation and translation methodology, *Evaluation and the Health Professions*, 29(1): 126–53.

Greene, J. (1993) Qualitative program evaluation, in N. Denzin and Y. Lincoln (eds) *Handbook of Qualitative Research*. London: Sage, pp. 530–44.

Greene, S., Reiter, K., Kilpatrick, K., Leatherman. S., Somers, S. and Hamblin, A. (2008) Searching for a business case for quality in Medicaid managed care, *Health Care Management Review*, 3(4): 350–60.

Greenhalgh, T., Humphrey, C., Hughes, J., Macfarlane, F., Butler, C., Connell, P. and Pawson, R. (2008) *The Modernisation Initiative Independent Evaluation: Final Report*. London: University College London. Available at: http://www.ucl.ac.uk/openlearning/research.htm (accessed 30 March 2009).

Greenhalgh, T., Humphrey, C., Hughes, J., Macfarlane, F., Butler, C. and Pawson, R. (2009) How do you modernize a health service? A realist evaluation of whole-scale transformation in London, *The Milbank Quarterly*, 87(2): 391–416.

Greenhalgh, T. and Peacock, R. (2005) Effectiveness and efficiency of search methods in systematic reviews of complex evidence: audit of primary sources, *BMJ*. Online. doi:10.1136/bmj.38636.593461.68.

Greenhalgh, T., Robert, G., Bate, P., Kyriakidou, O., Macfarlane, F. and Peacock, R. (2004) How to spread good ideas: a systematic review of the literature on diffusion, dissemination and sustainability of innovations in health service delivery and organisation. National Co-ordinating Centre for NHS Service Delivery and Organisation Research & Development (NCCSDO) 1–424. Available at: www.sdo.lshtm.ac.uk (accessed 2 January 2014).

Greenhalgh, T. and Russell, J. (2010) Why do evaluations of ehealth programs fail? an alternative set of guiding principles, *PLOS Medicine*, 1 November, 7(11), e1000360.

Greenhalgh, T., Stramer, K., Bratan, T., Byrne, E., Russell, J., Hinder, S. and Potts, H. (2010a) *The Devil's in the Detail: Final Report of the Independent Evaluation of the Summary Care Record and Health Space Programmes*. London: University College London.

Greenhalgh, T., Stramer, K., Bratan, T., Byrne, E., Russell, J. and Potts, H. (2010b) Adoption and non-adoption of a shared electronic summary record in England: a mixed-method case study, *BMJ*, 340:c3111. doi:10.1136/bmj.c3111.

Grimshaw, J.M., Thomas, R., MacLennan, G., Fraser, C.R. Ramsay, L., et al. (2004) Effectiveness and efficiency of guideline dissemination and implementation strategies, *Health Technology Assessment*, 8(6): iii–72.

Guba, E. and Lincoln, Y. (1989) *Fourth Generation Evaluation*. London: Sage.

Gustafson, D., Brennan, P. and Hawkins, R. (eds) (2007) *Investing in E-Health: What It Takes to Sustain Consumer Health Informatics*. New York: Springer.

Guyatt, G.H., Oxman, A.D., Vist, G.E., Kunz, R., Falck-Ytter, Y. and Alonso-Coello, P., et al. (2008) GRADE: an emerging consensus on rating quality of evidence and strength of recommendations, *BMJ*, 336: 924–6.

Harper, J. (1986) Measuring performance: a new approach, *Hospital and Health Services Review*, January, 26–8.

Hart, E. and Bond, M. (1996) *Action Research for Health and Social Care*. Milton Keynes: Open University Press.

Hawe, P., Degeling, D. and Hall, J. (1990) *Evaluating Health Promotion*. Artamon, Australia: MacLennan & Petty.

Hawe, P., King, L., Noort, M., Jordens, C. and Lloyd, P. (2000) Indicators to help with capacity building in health promotion, NSW Health Department. Available at: http://www0.health.nsw.gov.au/pubs/2000/pdf/capbuild.pdf (accessed 2 January 2014).

Hawe, P., et al. (2004) Methods for exploring implementation variation and local context within a cluster randomised community intervention trial, *Journal of Epidemiology of Community Health*, 58(9): 788–93.

Hawe, P. and Potvin, L. (2009) What is population health intervention research? *Canadian Journal of Public Health*, 100(1): Suppl.: 18–14.

Haycox, A. (1994) A methodology for estimating the costs and benefits of health promotion, *Health Promotion International*, 9(7): 5–11.

HealthyPeople.gov (2011) Healthy People 2020, Determinants of Health. Washington DC: US Department of Health and Human Services. Available at http://www.healthypeople.gov/2020/about/DOHAbout.aspx (accessed 29 June 2011).

Helfrich, C., Li, Y., Sharp, N. and Sales, A. (2009) Organizational readiness to change assessment (ORCA): development of an instrument based on the Promoting Action on Research in Health Services (PARIHS) framework. *Implementation Science*, 4: 38. doi:10.1186/1748-5908-4-38.

HERG (1996) *Economic Evaluation in Healthcare Research and Development: Undertake It Early and Often*. Uxbridge: Health Economics Research Group, Brunel University.

Hibbard, J., Stockard, J., Mahoney, R. and Tusler, M. (2004) Development of the Patient Activation Measure (PAM): conceptualizing and measuring activation in patients and consumers, *Health Services Research*, 39: 4, Part I.

Hickson, G., Clayton, E., Entman, S., Miller, C., Githens, P., Whetten-Goldstein, K. and Sloan, F. (1994) Obstetricians' prior malpractice experience and patients' satisfaction with care. *JAMA*, 272(20): 1583–7.

Hickson, G.B. and Pichert, J.W. (2007) Identifying and intervening with high-malpractice-risk physicians to reduce claims, *Physician Insurer*, 4: 29–36.

HONF (2013) Health On the Net Foundation Standards for Web Sites. Available at: www.HealthOnNet.org (accessed 21 November 2013).

Hospital Compare (2014) *Medicare Hospital Comparisons*. Washington, DC: CMS. Available at: http://www.medicare.gov/hospitalcompare/search.html?AspxAutoDetectCookieSupport=1 (accessed 4 January 2014).

Hunter, D. (1992) Rationing dilemmas in health care, NAHA & T Paper 8, Birmingham.

Hvitfeldt, H., Carli, C.A., Nelson, E.C., et al. (2009) Feed-forward systems for patient participation and provider support: adoption results from the original US context to Sweden and beyond, *Quality Management in Health Care*, 18: 247–56.

Inamdar, N., Kaplan, R.S. and Bower, M. (2002) Applying the balanced scorecard in healthcare provider organizations, *Journal of Healthcare Management*, 47(3): 179–95.

IOM (Institute of Medicine) (2007) *The Learning Healthcare System*. Workshop Series Summary. Institute of Medicine Roundtable on Evidence-Based Medicine. Available at: http://www.nap.edu/catalog/11903.html.

IOM (Institute of Medicine) (2010) *The Healthcare Imperative: Lowering Costs and Improving Outcomes*. Workshop Series Summary. Washington, DC: The National Academies Press. Available at: http://www.nap.edu/catalog/12750.html.

Jackson, C. (1997) *Evaluation of the Exercise by Prescription Programme*. Harrogate: North Yorkshire Health Authority.

Janzen, J., Buurman, B., Spanjaard, L., et al. (2013 Reduction of unnecessary use of indwelling urinary catheters, *BMJ Quality and Safety*; 22: 681–8.

JC (Joint Commission) (2013) *About Our Standards*. Oak Brook, IL: The Joint Commission. Available at: http://www.jointcommission.org/standards_information/standards.aspx (accessed 4 January 2014).

JCSEE (US Joint Committee on Standards for Educational Evaluation) (1994) *The Programme Evaluation Standards: How to Assess Evaluations of Educational Programs*, 2nd edn. Thousand Oaks, CA: Sage.

Kaplan, H., Provost, L., Froehle, C. and Margolis, P. (2011) The Model for Understanding Success in Quality (MUSIQ): building a theory of context in healthcare quality improvement, *BMJ Quality and Safety*. doi:10.1136/bmjqs-2011-000010.

Keen, J. (1994) Evaluation: informing the future not living in the past, in J. Keen (ed.) *Information Management in Health Services*. Buckingham: Open University Press.

Keen, J. and Packwood, T. (1995) Qualitative research: case study evaluation, *BMJ*, 311: 444–6.

Kessler, R. and Glasgow, R. (2011) A proposal to speed translation of healthcare research into practice dramatic change is needed, *American Journal of Preventative Medicine*, 40(6): 637–44.

Kilo, C. (1998) A framework for collaborative improvement: lessons from the Institute for Healthcare Improvement's Breakthrough Series, *Quality Management in Health Care*, 6(4): 1–13.

King, D.K., Glasgow, R.E. and Leeman-Castillo, B.A. (2010) Reaiming RE-AIM: using the model to plan, implement, and evaluate the effects of environmental change approaches to enhancing population health, *American Journal of Public Health*, 100(1): 2076–84.

King, R. and He, J. (2006) A meta-analysis of the technology acceptance model, *Information & Management*, 43: 740–55.

Kirkland, K.B., Homa, K.A., Lasky, R.A., et al. (2012) Impact of a hospital-wide hand hygiene initiative on healthcare-associated infections: results of an interrupted time series, *BMJ Quality and Safety*. Online First: 24 July 2012. doi: 10.1136/bmjqs-2012-000800.

Klein, H.K. and Myers, M.D. (1999) A set of principles for conducting and evaluating interpretive field studies in information systems, *MIS Quarterly*, 23: 67–93.

Kolata, G. (2014) Method of study is criticized in group's health policy tests, *New York Times*, 2 February 2014. Available at: http://www.nytimes.com/2014/02/03/health/effort-to-test-health-policies-is-criticized-for-study-tactics.html (accessed 6 February 2014).

Landon, B.E., Normand, S.-L.T., Blumenthal, D. and Daley, J. (2003) Physician clinical performance assessment: prospects and barriers, *JAMA*, 290: 1183–9.

Langley, G.J., Nolan, K.M., Nolan, T.W., Norman, C.N. and Provost, L.P. (1996) *The Improvement*

Guide: A Practical Approach to Enhancing Organizational Performance. San Francisco: Jossey-Bass.

Leatherman, S., Berwick, D., Iles, D., Lewin, L. S., Davidoff, F., Nolan, T. and Bisognano, M. (2003) The business case for quality: case studies and an analysis, *Health Affairs*, 22: 17–30.

Lehmann, H. and Ohno-Machado, L. (2011) Evaluation of informatics systems: beyond RCTs and beyond the hospital, *Journal of American Medical Informatics Association*, 18(2): 110–11.

Lincoln, Y. and Guba, E. (1985) *Naturalistic Inquiry*, Newbury Park, CA: Sage.

Liu, J.L. and Wyatt, J.C. (2011) The case for randomized controlled trials to assess the impact of clinical information systems, *Journal of American Medical Informatics Association*, 18:173e80.

Lockwood, F. (1994) *Exercise by Prescription in York and Selby*. Harrogate: North Yorkshire Health Authority.

Lorig, K., Chastain, R., Ung, E., Shoor, S. and Holman, H. (1989) Development and evaluation of a scale to measure perceived self-efficacy in people with arthritis, *Arthritis & Rheumatology*, 32: 37–44.

Magid, D.J., Estabrooks, P.A., Brand, D.W., et al. (2004) Translating patient safety research into clinical practice. advances in patient safety: from research to implementation. Agency for Healthcare Research and Quality, National Institutes of Health. Available at: http://www.ahrq.gov/qual/advances (accessed 4 January 2014).

Mann, C. (2003) Observational research methods: research design II: cohort, cross sectional, and case-control studies, *Emergency Medicine Journal*, 20: 54–60.

Marks, S., et al. (1980) Ambulatory surgery in an HMO, *Medical Care*, 18, 127–46.

Marshall, M. and Øvretveit, J. (2011) Can we save money by improving quality? *BMJ Quality and Safety*, 20: 293–6.

Mauskopf, P., et al. (2007) Principles of good practice for budget impact analysis: report of the ISPOR Task Force on Good Research Practices: budget impact, *Analysis Value in Health*, 10(5): 336–47.

Mays, N., Pope, C. and Popay, J. (2005) Systematically reviewing qualitative and quantitative evidence to inform management and policy-making in the health field, *Journal of Health Services Research and Policy*, 10(3): Suppl.: 1: 6–20.

McGaughey, J., et al. (2007) Outreach and early warning systems (EWS) for the prevention of intensive care admission and death of critically ill adult patients on general hospital wards, *Cochrane Database Systems Review*, July 18 (3).

Mercer, S., DeVinney, B., Fine, L., Green, L. and Dougherty, D. (2007) Study designs for effectiveness and translation research identifying trade-offs, *American Journal of Preventative Medicine*, 33(2): 139–54.

Michie, S., Fixsen, D., Grimshaw, J. and Eccles, M. (2009) Specifying and reporting complex behaviour change interventions: the need for a scientific method, *Implementation Science*, 4: 40. doi:10.1186/1748-5908-4-40.

Moore, S. (2012) *Realist Evaluation: What Works, for Whom, in What Circumstances*. Veterans' Health Administration Cyber seminar series. Available at: http://www.hsrd.research.va.gov/cyberseminars/catalog-archive.cfm#.UrXMd2RAQkY (accessed 22 December 2013).

MRC (2000) *A Framework for Development and Evaluation of RCTs for Complex Interventions to Improve Health*. London: Medical Research Council. Available at: www.mrc.ac.uk/pdf-mrc_cpr.pdf (accessed January 2004).

Nazareth, I., Freemantle, N., Duggan, C., Mason, J. and Haines, A. (2002) Evaluation of a complex intervention for changing professional behavior: the Evidence Based Out Reach (EBOR) trial, *Journal of Health Services Research & Policy*, 7(4): 230–8.

NCQA (2013) *HEDIS and Performance Measurement*. Available at: http://www.ncqa.org/HEDISQualityMeasurement.aspx (accessed 21 December 2013).

NHS (2014) *Choices, Comparing Hospitals, GPs and Dentists*. Available at: http://www.nhs.uk/aboutNHSChoices/professionals/developments/Pages/NHSChoicesdatasets.aspx (accessed 4 January 2014).

Nightingale, F. (1863) *Notes on Hospitals*, 3rd edn. London: Longman, Green, Longman, Roberts and Green.

NIII (2011) Return on investment (ROI) calculator. Available at: http://www.institute.nhs.uk/quality_and_service_improvement_tools/quality_and_service_improvement_tools.

NIII (2014) *Balanced Scorecard*. UK NHS Institute for Innovation and Improvement. Available at: http://www.institute.nhs.uk/quality_and_service_improvement_tools/quality_and_service_improvement_tools/balanced_scorecard.html (accessed 4 January 2014).

Norton, W., Cannon, J., Schall, M. and Mittman, B. (2012) A stakeholder-driven agenda for advancing the science and practice of scale-up and spread in health, *Implementation Science*, 7:118. Available at: http://www.implementationscience.com/content/7/1/118.

NYT (2014) Method of Study is Criticized in Group's Health Policy Tests, *New York Times*, Available at: http://www.nytimes.com/2014/02/03/health/effort-to-test-health-policies-is-crticized-for-study-tactics.html (accessed 6 February 2014).

Nuti, S., Seghieri, C. and Vainieri, M.J. (2012) Assessing the effectiveness of a performance evaluation system in the public health care sector: some novel evidence from the Tuscany region experience, *Journal of Management and Governance*. doi: 10.1007/s10997-012-9218-5.

Ogrinc, G., Mooney, S., Estrada, C., et al. (2008) The SQUIRE (Standards for QUality Improvement Reporting Excellence) guidelines for quality improvement reporting: explanation and elaboration, *Quality and Safety in Health Care*, 17: i13–i32. doi: 10.1136/qshc.2008.029058.

Olsen, J. and Donaldson, C. (1993) Willingness to pay for public sector health care programmes in Northern Norway, HERU Discussion Paper, University of Aberdeen.

Øvretveit, J. (1992) *Health Service Quality*. Oxford: Blackwell Scientific Press.

Øvretveit, J. (1993) *Coordinationg Community Care: Multidisciplinary Teams and Care Management in Health and Social Services*. Milton Keynes: Open University Press.

Øvretveit, J. (1996) Quality in health promotion, *Health Promotion International*, 11(1): 55–62.

Øvretveit, J. (1998) *Evaluating Health Interventions*. Milton Keynes: Open University Press.

Øvretveit, J. (2000) A team quality improvement sequence for complex problems (TQIS), *Quality in Health Care*, 8: 1–7.

Øvretveit, J. (2002) *Action Evaluation of Health Programmes and Change*. Oxford: Radcliffe Medical Press.

Øvretveit, J. (2011a) Widespread focused improvement: lessons from international health for spreading specific improvements to health services in high-income countries, *International Journal of Quality in Health Care*, 23: 239–46.

Øvretveit, J. (2011b) Implementing, sustaining, and spreading quality improvement, in Joint Commission Resources, *From Office to Front Line: Essential Issues for Health Care Leaders*, 2nd edn. Oak Brook, IL: Joint Commission Resources, pp. 159–76.

Øvretveit, J. (2011c) *Does Clinical Coordination Improve Quality and Save Money? Summary*, Volume 1. London: The Health Foundation. Available at: www.health.org.uk; and http://public.me.com/johnovr.http://www.health.org.uk/publications/does-clinical-coordination-improve-quality-and-save-money/.

Øvretveit, J. (2012) *Do Changes to Patient–Provider Relationships Improve Quality and Save Money? A Review of Evidence about Value Improvements Made by Changing*

Communication, Collaboration and Support for Self-Care. London: The Health Foundation. Available at: www.health.org.uk.

Øvretveit, J. (2013) *Evaluating Complex Social Interventions and their Implementation:* vol. 1: *Challenges and Choices*. Sepulveda, CA: CIPRS, Veterans' Health Administration.

Øvretveit, J., Andreen-Sachs, M., Carlsson, J., Gustafsson, H., Lofgren, S., et al. (2012) Implementing organization and management innovations in Swedish healthcare: lessons from a comparison of 12 cases, *Journal of Health Organisation and Management*, 26(2): 237–7.

Øvretveit, J. and Aslaksen, A. (1999) *The Quality Journeys of Six Norwegian Hospitals*. Oslo, Norway: Norwegian Medical Association.

Øvretveit, J. and Gustafson, D. (2003) Evaluation of quality improvement programmes, *BMJ*, 326: 759–61.

Øvretveit, J., Keller, C., Hvitfeldt Forsberg, H., Essén, A., Lindblad, S. and Brommels, M. (2013) Continuous innovation: the development and use of the Swedish rheumatology register to improve the quality of arthritis care, *International Journal for Quality in Health Care*, 25(2). doi: 10.1093/intqhc/mzt002.

Øvretveit, J. and Mäntyranta, T. (2007) *Research Informed Professional Practice for Rohto Interventions to Improve Prescribing*. Helsinki: Centre for Pharmacotherapy Development.

Øvretveit, J., Scott, T., Rundall, T., Shortell, S. and Brommels, M. (2007) Implementation of electronic medical records in hospitals: two case studies, *Health Policy*, 84: 181–90.

Owen, J. and Rodgers, P. (1999) *Program Evaluation: Forms and Approaches*. London: Sage.

Ozcan, Y. (2013) *Health Care Benchmarking and Performance Evaluation*. New York: Springer.

Patton, M.Q. (1997) *Utilisation-Focused Evaluation: The New Century*, 3rd edn. London: Sage.

Pawson, R. and Tilley, N. (1997) *Realistic Evaluation*. London: Sage.

Pearson, J.F., Brownstein, C.A. and Brownstein, J.S. (2011) Potential for electronic health records and online social networking to redefine medical research, *Clinical Chemistry*, 57, 196–204.

Penchon, D. (2014) *The Good Indicators Guide: Understanding How to Use and Choose Indicators*. NHS Institute for Innovation and Improvement. Available at: www.institute.nhs.uk (accessed 4 January 2014).

Peters, D.H., Noor, A.A., Singh, L.P., Kakar, F.K., Hansen, P.M. and Burnham, G. (2007) A balanced scorecard for health services in Afghanistan, *Bulletin of World Health Organization*, 85: 146–51.

PHAB (2014) *Public Health Accreditation Board Standards*. Available at: http://www.phaboard.org./ (accessed 2 January 2014).

Poon, E., Cusack, C. and McGowan, J. (2009) Evaluating healthcare information technology outside of academia: observations from the National Resource Center for Healthcare Information Technology at the Agency for Healthcare Research and Quality, *Journal of American Medical Informatics Association*, 16(5): 631–6.

Potvin, L., Haddad, S. and Frohlich, K.L. (2001) *Beyond Process and Outcome Evaluation: A Comprehensive Approach for Evaluating Health Promotion Programmes*. WHO Regional Publications European Series (92): 45–62.

PPACA (2010) Patient Protection and Affordable Care Act of 2010, Public Law 111–148, U.S. Statutes at Large 124 573 (2010).

Preskill, H. and Jones, N. (2012) *A Practical Guide for Engaging Stakeholders in Developing Evaluation Questions*. Foundation Strategy Group. Available at: http://trasi.foundationcenter.org/browse.php.

Pronovost, P.J., Berenholtz, S.M., Goeschel, C., et al. (2008) Improving patient safety in intensive care units in Michigan. *Journal of Critical Care*, 23(2): 207–21.

Puska, P., Nissinen, A. and Tuomilehto, J. (1985) The community-based strategy to prevent coronary heart disease: conclusions for the ten years of the North Karelia Projects, *Annual Review of Public Health*, 6: 147–93.

Puska, P., Tuomilehto, J., Nissinen, A., et al. (eds) (1995) *The North Karelia Project. 20 Y Results and Experiences*. Helsinki: Helsinki University Press.

Puska, P., Tuomilehto, J., Salonen, J., et al. (1981) Community control of cardiovascular diseases: The North Karelia Project, in *Evaluation of a Comprehensive Community Programme for Control of Cardiovascular Diseases in North Karelia, Finland, 1972–1977*. Copenhagen: WHO Regional Office for Europe.

RCGP (2013) *The RCGP Guide to the Revalidation of General Practitioners*. London: Royal College of General Practitioners. Available at: http://www.rcgp.org.uk/revalidation-and-cpd/~/media/Files/Revalidation-and-CPD/Revalidation/Guidance-for-GPs/1-Guide%20to%20Revalidation%20Version%208_FINAL.ashx (accessed 20 March 2013).

RE-AIM (2014) The Reach Effectiveness Adoption Implementation Maintenance (RE-AIM) framework. Available at: http://re-aim.org/ (accessed 2 January 2014).

Redfern, S., Christian, S. and Norman, I. (2002) Evaluating change in health care practice: lessons from three studies, *Journal of Evaluation in Clinical Practice*, 9(2): 239–49.

Reiter, K.L., Kilpatrick, K.E., Greene, S.B., Lohr, K.N. and Leatherman, S. (2007) How to develop a business case for quality, *International Journal for Quality in Health Care*, 19: 50–5.

Research Utilization Support and Health (2009) Toolbox and Resources. Available at: http://www.researchutilization.org/learnru/welcome2ru/, and http://www.researchutilization.org/matrix/resources/index.html (accessed 4 January 2014).

Richardson, J. (1992) Cost-utility analyses in health care: present status and future issues, in J. Daly, I. McDonald, and E. Willis (eds) *Researching Health Care: Designs, Dilemmas, Disciplines*. London: Routledge, pp. 21–44.

Riley, W., Glasgow, R., Etheredge, L. and Abernethy, A. (2013) Rapid, responsive, relevant (R3) research: a call for a rapid learning health research enterprise, *Clinical and Translational Medicine*, 2:10. Available at: http://www.clintransmed.com/content/2/1/10.

Robson, C. (1993) *Real World Research*, Oxford: Blackwell.

Rootman, I., Goodstadt, M., Potvin, L. and Springett, J. (1997) Toward a framework for health promotion evaluation, background paper for the WHO-EURO Working Group on Health Promotion, Copenhagen: WHO.

Rootman, I. and McQueen, D. (eds) (1997) *Evaluating Health Promotion Approaches*. Copenhagen: WHO.

Royston, C., Lansdown, M. and Brought, W. (1994) Teaching laparoscopic surgery: the need for guidelines, *BMJ*, 308(6935): 1023–5.

Rubenstein, L., Chaney, E., Ober, S., Felker, B., Sherman, S., Lanto, A. and Vivell, S. (2010) Using evidence-based quality improvement methods for translating depression collaborative care research into practice, *Families, Systems, & Health*, 28(2): 91–113. doi: 10.1037/a0020302.

Rubenstein, L.V., Meredith, L.S., et al. (2006) Impacts of evidence-based quality improvement on depression in primary care: a randomized experiment, *Journal of General International Medicine*, 21(10): 1027–35. Epub 2006 July 7.

Rycroft-Malone, J., Wilkinson, J., Burton, C., et al. (2011) Implementing health research through academic and clinical partnerships: a realistic evaluation of the Collaborations for Leadership in Applied Health Research and Care (CLAHRC), *Implementation Science*, 6: 74. Available at: http://www.implementationscience.com/content/6/1/74.

Sackett, D., Rosenberg, W., Gray, J., Haynes, R. and Scott-Richardson, W. (1996) Evidence-based medicine: what it is and what it isn't. *BMJ*, 312, pp. 71–2.

Scales, D.C., Dainty, K., Hales, B., et al. (2011) A multifaceted intervention for quality improvement in a network of intensive care units: a cluster randomized trial, *JAMA*, 305: 363–72.

Schouten, L., Hulscher, M., van Everdingen, J., Huijsman, R. and Grol, R. (2008) Evidence for the impact of quality improvement collaboratives: systematic review, *BMJ*, 336: 1491–4.

Schulz, K.F., Altman, D.G., Moher, D. for the CONSORT Group (2010) CONSORT 2010 Statement: updated guidelines for reporting parallel group randomised trial, *BMJ*, 340: 698–702. doi: 10.1136/bmj.c332.

Scriven, M. (1991) *Evaluation Thesaurus*. London: Sage.

Shadish, W., Cook, T. and Leviton, L. (1991) *Foundations of Programme Evaluation: Theories of Practice*. London: Sage.

Shekelle, P.G., Pronovost, P.J., Wachter, R.M., Taylor, S.L., Dy, S., Foy, R., Øvretveit, J., et al. (2010) *Assessing the Evidence for Context-Sensitive Effectiveness and Safety of Patient Safety Practices: Developing Criteria*. Rockville, MD: Agency for Healthcare Research and Quality, AHRQ Publication No. 11-0006-EF Contract No. HHSA-2902009-10001C. Available at: http://www.ahrq.gov/qual/contextsensitive/.

SMAC (Standing Medical Advisory Committee) (1990) *Blood Cholesterol Screening: The Cost Effectiveness of Opportunistic Cholesterol Testing*. London: SMAC.

Smith, J. (1992) Ethics and health care rationing, *Journal of Management in Medicine*, 89: 26–8.

Speroff, T. and O'Connor, G.T. (2004) Study designs for PDSA quality improvement research. *Quality Management in Health Care*, 13(1): 17–32.

SSSSG (1994) Randomised trial of cholesterol lowering in 4444 patients with coronary heart disease, *Lancet*, 344: 1383–9.

Stetler, C.B., Damschroder, L.J., Helfrich, C.D., et al. (2011) A guide for applying a revised version of the PARIHS framework for implementation, *Implementation Science*, 6: 99. PMID: 21878092.

Steventon, A., Bardsley, M., Billings, J., et al. (2013) Effect of telehealth on use of secondary care and mortality according to routine operational data sets: findings from the Whole Systems Demonstrator cluster randomised trial, *BMJ* 344. doi 10.1136/bmj.e3874.

Stiefel, M. and Nolan, K. (2012) *A Guide to Measuring the Triple Aim: Population Health, Experience of Care, and Per Capita Cost*. IHI Innovation Series White Paper. Cambridge, MA: Institute for Healthcare Improvement. Available at: www.IHI.org.

Stoop, S., Heathfield, H., de Mul, M. and Berg, M. (2004) Evaluation of patient care information systems: theory and practice, in Evaluating ICT Applications in Health Care, thesis, 25 Nov. Available at: http://hdl.handle.net/1765/7108 (accessed 23 November 2013).

TCWF (2014) *Why Not the Best?* Washington, DC: The Commonwealth Fund. Available at: http://www.whynotthebest.org (accessed 4 January 2014).

Tolley, K., Buck, D. and Godfrey, C. (1996) Health promotion and health economics, *Health Education Research*, 11(3): 361–4.

Tunis, S.R., Stryer, D.B. and Clancy, C.M. (2003) Practical clinical trials: increasing the value of clinical research for decision making in clinical and health policy, *JAMA*, 290: 1624–32.

UCH (2014) Appraisal for senior medical staff, University Hospitals of Southampton, UK. Available at: http://www.uhs.nhs.uk/Education/Informationforstaff/Doctors/Appraisalforseniormedicalstaff/AppraisalforSeniorMedicalStaff.aspx (accessed 4 January 2014).

UKIHI (UK Institute of Health Informatics) (2001) *Evaluation of Electronic Patient and Health Record Projects*. Winchester: ERDIP Programme, NHS Information Authority.

Van Deusen Lukas, C., Meterko, M., Mohr, D. and Nealon-Seibert, M. (2004) *The Implementation and Effectiveness of Advanced Clinic Access*. Veterans' Health Administration report.

Available at: http://www.colmr.research.va.gov/publications/reports/ACA_FullReport.pdf (accessed 6 February 2014).

Wagenaar, A.C. and Komro, K.A. (2011) *Natural Experiments: Design Elements for Optimal Causal Inference.* PHLR Methods Monograph Series. Philadelphia, PA: Temple University Press.

Walshe, K. and Shortell, S. (2004) What happens when things go wrong: how healthcare organisations deal with major failures in care, *Health Affairs*, 23(3): 103–11.

Waterman, H., Tillen, D., Dickson, R. and de Koning, K. (2001) Action research: a systematic review and guidance for assessment, *Health Technology Assessment*, 5: 23.

Waters, E., Doyle, J., Jackson, N., Howes, F., Brunton, G. and Oakley, A. (2006) Evaluating the effectiveness of public health interventions: the role and activities of the Cochrane Collaboration. *Journal of Epidemiology of Community Health*, 60: 285–9. doi:10.1136/jech.2003.015354.

Wheeler, D. (1993) *Understanding Variation*, Tennessee. SPC Press.

WHO (1981) *Health Programme Evaluation.* Geneva: World Health Organization.

Williams I. (2011) Organizational readiness for innovation in health care: some lessons from the recent literature, *Health Services Management Research* 24(4): 213–18.

Woodard, G., McLean, S., Green, K., Moore, M. and Williams, L. (2004) *Health Promotion Capacity Checklists: A Workbook for Individual, Organizational and Environmental Assessment.* Saskatchewan: Prairie Region Health Promotion Research Centre University of Saskatchewan Saskatoon. Available at: www.usask.ca/healthsci/che/prhprc/programs/finalworkbook.pdf (accessed 2 January 2014).

Yin, L. ([1989]) 1994) *Case Study Research: Design and Methods*, Beverly Hills, CA: Sage.

Yin, R. (1981) The case study: some answers. *Administrative Science Quarterly*, 26(1), 58–65.

Zapka, J., Valentine-Goins, K., Pebert, L. and Ockene, K. (2004) Translating efficacy research to effectiveness studies in practice: lessons from research to promote smoking cessation in community health centers, *Health Promotion Practice*, 5: 245–55.

Index

Made in the USA
Lexington, KY
02 June 2015